2

# The Entrepreneur® Diet

# The Entrepreneur®
# Diet

## The On-the-Go Plan for Fitness, Weight Loss and Healthy Living

## TOM WEEDE
Former Senior Editor of
*Men's Fitness* magazine

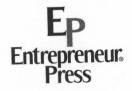

**Ep**
**Entrepreneur®**
**Press**

Editorial director: Jere L. Calmes
Cover design: Barry T. Kerrigan
Composition and production: Eliot House Productions

This publication is designed to provide accurate and authoritative information in regard to the subject matter covered. It is sold with the understanding that the publisher is not engaged in rendering legal, accounting, or other professional services. If legal advice or other expert assistance is required, the services of a competent professional person should be sought.

Exercise photos by Julia Cappelli
Back cover photo by Mary Kay Stein, Desert Light Photography

**Library of Congress Cataloging-in-Publication Data**
Weede, Tom.
    The entrepreneur diet: the on-the-go plan for fitness, weight loss and healthy living/by Tom Weede.
        p.    cm.
    ISBN 1-59918-060-X (alk. paper)
    1. Businesspeople—Health and hygiene. 2. Businesspeople—Nutrition. 3. Exercise. I. Title.
RA777.63.W44 2007
613.2'5—dc22                                                    2006023691

Printed in Canada

12 11 10 09 08 07

10 9 8 7 6 5 4 3 2 1

# Contents

PART II

*Start-Up*

PART III
## *Building Your Body's Equity*

PART IV

*Guaranteeing Your
Return on Investment*

# The Entrepreneur Diet Advisory Board

**Steven Knope, M.D.**                    www.conciergemedicinemd.com

Dr. Knope is a board-certified internist and sports medicine expert practicing in Tucson, Arizona. He graduated with honors in internal medicine from Cornell University Medical College and completed his residency training at UCLA. A highly regarded national speaker on the subjects of obesity, fitness, and exercise, he has served as chief of medicine, chairman of the Department of Medicine and director of the ICU in the Carondelet health system in Tucson. Dr. Knope also has acted as the official internist for the Colorado Rockies baseball team during spring training and has served on the editorial board of the American College of Sports Medicine's Health and Fitness Journal. A four-time Ironman triathlon finisher and third degree black belt in Kenpo Karate, Dr. Knope is the author of *The Body/Mind Connection: Exploring the Undeniable Power of Strength.*

**Don Powell, Ph.D.**                         www.healthylife.com

Dr. Powell is the president and CEO of the American Institute for Preventive Medicine, a Farmington Hills, Michigan, company that provides health management and wellness programs for more than 12,000 corporations, hospitals, unions, colleges, and government agencies. He has written many journal articles in the field of health promotion and is the author of *Healthier at Home* and *A Year of Health Hints*. He has also written a nationally syndicated newspaper column and articles for *Shape* magazine. Dr. Powell, a clinical psychologist, has won numerous awards for his work, including those from the President's Council on Physical Fitness and Sports, Department of Health and Human Services, Centers for Disease Control and Prevention, U.S. Jaycees, and the State of Michigan. He is a member of the U.S. government's "Healthy People 2010" project, which has set the nation's health goals for the beginning of the 21st century.

**Tyler Wallace**                                    www.nasm.org

Wallace is director of clinical services for the National Academy of Sports Medicine and a NASM performance-enhancement specialist and corrective-exercise specialist. He has trained and rehabilitated hundreds of professional, Olympic, collegiate, and high school athletes. He and NASM are currently in a revolutionary sports-medicine and performance-enhancement partnership with the Phoenix Suns in which they implement an integrated assessment process, leading to corrective-exercise, injury-prevention and performance-enhancement programs and techniques with impressive results.

**Michael G. Goldsby, Ph.D.**                www.bsu.edu/entrepreneurship

Dr. Goldsby is the Stoops Distinguished Professor of Entrepreneurship in the Department of Marketing and Management at the Miller College of Business at Ball State University. He is a nationally recognized expert on the links between health and entrepreneurial success. He has published research in the *Journal of Managerial Psychology, Eastern Economic Journal, Management Decision, Teaching Business Ethics*, and the *Journal of Legal Studies Education*. He is a member of the Academy of Management, International Association of Business and Society, Southern Management Association, Midwest Academy of Management, USASBE, and Society for Business Ethics. He has a doctorate in strategic studies in management from Virginia Tech, a master's degree in economics from Indiana State University, and a bachelor's degree in business economics and public policy from Indiana University.

**Kathy Wise, R.D.**                                    www.nutrawise.com

Wise is a nutrition consultant, wellness coach, speaker, and member of the executive board of the American Dietetic Association's Nutrition Entrepreneurs Practice Group. A registered dietitian, she has extensive experience in creating nutrition programs for hospitals, corporations, and individuals. She provides nutritional consulting services for restaurants, chefs, grocery stores, companies and families. A frequent speaker on nutrition and wellness, Wise has appeared on radio and television programs and is often quoted in the press. In 1993, she established Wise Nutrition Concepts Inc., to help people achieve and maintain good patterns of nutrition for life-long well-being. She separates the fads from the facts and gives professional support to people in the process of achieving a healthier lifestyle.

**Chad Luethje**                                    www.redmountainspa.com

Luethje is the executive chef at the Red Mountain Spa in St. George, Utah. He has more than 20 years of experience with some of the top resorts in the country, including Teton Mountain Lodge in Jackson Hole, Wyoming; Cedar Breaks Lodge in Brian Head, Utah; Enchantment Resort in Sedona, Arizona; and Loews Ventana Canyon Resort and Westin La Paloma Resort & Spa in Tucson, Arizona. Raised by health-conscious vegetarian parents, Luethje learned early to prefer and appreciate a healthy lifestyle. In addition to his chef's duties at Red Mountain, he works one-on-one with guests to create menu plans and provide healthy recipe alternatives.

**Paul Robbins**                                    www.athletesperformance.com

Robbins is a consultant on cardiovascular exercise to the National Academy of Sports Medicine. He is a metabolic specialist with Athletes' Performance in Tempe, Arizona, which includes doing research development with three major universities. He is also the president and owner of Cardio2Tech, a metabolic education, training, and installation company. He has published articles for *Shape, Fitness Management,* NASM, and PTontheNET.com, and in multiple research journals. Some of his metabolic clients include Navy SEALs and Army Rangers, as well as the Miami Heat, Phoenix Coyotes, Los Angeles Kings, Major League baseball players, elite tri-athlete clubs and health clubs throughout the United States.

**Rieva Lesonsky**     www.entrepreneur.com

Lesonsky is the editorial director of *Entrepreneur* magazine and senior vice president at Entrepreneur Media Inc. Under her editorial eye, *Entrepreneur* has become the nation's leading authority for and about entrepreneurs. Lesonsky wrote the best-selling book *Start Your Own Business,* currently in its third edition, and has co-authored several other books about how to start and grow a small business. Lesonsky served on the Small Business Administration's National Advisory Council for six years. The SBA also honored her as a Small Business Media Advocate and a Woman in Business Advocate. For five consecutive years, she was named one of the Top 100 Most Influential Journalists by *Business News Reporter*. A nationally recognized speaker and expert on small business and entrepreneurship, Lesonsky has appeared on numerous national TV programs, including *The Today Show, Martha Stewart, Good Morning America,* and *Oprah.*

# Acknowledgments

I am indebted to the entrepreneurs who shared their insights into how their healthy lifestyles have contributed to their business success. Their real-world experience brought meaning to the book's advice. Members of the advisory board—Michael G. Goldsby, Ph.D.; Steven Knope, M.D.; Rieva Lesonsky; chef Chad Luethje; Don Powell, Ph.D.; Paul Robbins; Tyler Wallace; and Kathy Wise, RD—gave generously of their time and considerable expertise to provide invaluable input. Their extensive knowledge in the fields of health and fitness as well as business gave me access to cutting-edge information. Kathy Wise's original meal plan is central to the book's theme and her nutrition know-how helped tremendously in navigating a complex subject. Thanks also to Margaret Moore of Wellcoaches, who provided her insights on how to encourage long-lasting change. The experts at the National Academy of Sports Medicine (NASM) freely shared their innovative approaches to fitness, which are helping countless people have a better quality of life. The academy's staff also made available exercise information that added significantly to the book, and thank you to Scott Lucett, M.S., and Brian Sutton, M.A. for coordinating that effort.

Editors Jere Calmes and Karen Thomas at Entrepreneur Press provided encouragement, guidance, and insights throughout the writing process, with Jere generating the original idea for the book. I am grateful for the confidence they showed in me during this project. Karen Billipp at Eliot House Productions greatly improved the manuscript with a sharp eye for substance, editing detail, and layout design. Her tireless efforts were indispensable. Leanne Harvey and Stephanie Singer at Entrepreneur Press have worked hard to get out the messages of this book. JoAnn Clupper, with coordination by Anne Sommers of the Temp Connection, skillfully transcribed numerous interviews.

And thank you to my wife, Adrienne, and my parents, Robert and Vivian, who gave valuable editing advice, suggestions, and unflinching moral support.

# Preface

After seven years of working as a software developer for a Wall Street company, Terri Alpert decided to follow the call of her entrepreneurial spirit. "I've always been an entrepreneur at heart," she says. "I knew that ultimately I would have my own business."

So in 1993, she took the plunge and launched a consumer catalog business, using just $8,000 in initial funding. "I started with the goal of seeing if there was a real business I could create from $10,000 or less," she says. "Then things evolved from there."

Today, Alpert runs three consumer catalogs, including PCD's *Cooking Enthusiast* and the fast-growing *Uno Alla Volta*, with total revenues of more than $15 million, 50 year-round employees, and up to 150 seasonal employees.

And yet, with so much of her attention on the business in the early years, Alpert let something slip: a focus on her own well-being. Her weight climbed and was exacerbated by the birth of her two children. "I was getting backaches," she recalls. "I was generally not feeling well and didn't have the energy to either deal with the business or enjoy life."

It's understandable, really. With the laserlike focus it takes to build a successful company, it's not a surprise that an entrepreneur's own health could move 10 or 20 places down the priority list. But Alpert came to a turning point, realizing that she had to bring balance back into her life and take care of herself—before she could take care of the business. "Otherwise I wouldn't have the emotional or physical wherewithal to do what I needed to do," she says. Beginning in 1999, she made a vow to make her health and fitness a high priority. "Ever since then, I've been going to the gym five days a week," she says. "I've also made a full lifestyle change with food intake."

She's now 30 pounds lighter overall—actually, Alpert has lost at least 50 pounds of fat, having added muscle to her body. "I did it very, very slowly but consistently," she says. "Now I recognize the person in the mirror again as being the 'me' I remember and not the 'me' of the early years of the business."

For years, Alpert *had* thought she couldn't afford to take time away from her business to eat right and go to the gym. "That was a mistake," she says. "I believe my business has benefited considerably from my general happiness and my ability to manage stress better—much better."

◆ ◆ ◆ ◆ ◆

For Brian Scudamore, the road to entrepreneurial success started at a McDonald's drive-through, of all places. Needing a way to pay his college tuition so he could study business, Scudamore was struck with inspiration under the Golden Arches. "There was this beat-up old pickup truck in front of me, with plywood sides built up," he recalls. "I just looked at the truck and said: 'Hey, there's my ticket. Go haul junk.'"

Sixteen years and lots of junk pickups later—he did the driving for the first six years—Scudamore's idea for earning college cash has become a $72 million business. Known as 1-800-GOT-JUNK?, the company now boasts more than 200 franchises in 38 U.S. states, four Canadian provinces, Australia, and Britain. In 2005, Scudamore was a finalist for Ernst & Young's Entrepreneur of the Year Award.

But the years devoted to his business brought an unwelcome side effect: an expanded waistline—something that increasingly bothered Scudamore. "I just got to a point where I said, 'You know, I'm not feeling very good about myself,'" he recalls. And so, after years of downplaying his own health, Scudamore—like Alpert—finally resolved to do something about it and he started exercising and watching the foods he was eating.

Walking to and from the office with his dog Grizzly, Scudamore lost 34 pounds. But, as it turns out, the 36-year-old CEO didn't just drop the weight. With his newfound fitness, he gained a renewed energy that directly affected his business performance. "I'm much more focused at work," he says. "Mentally, I'm much stronger."

Today, his workout routine includes weight training, and he's eating more whole foods instead of fast food. That fast-food habit of his early business days is firmly in the past. "I'm making healthier choices and sticking to them," he says. "And I'm just feeling better for it."

Despite the demands of running his company, Scudamore has found the time to train for one of the largest running events in Canada, the 10K Vancouver Sun Run, and his fitness enthusiasm has taken hold in the office. "There's an even larger group of us this year planning on doing it as a company event. So we'll all be wearing our 'Powered by Junk?' running shirts."

◆ ◆ ◆ ◆ ◆

Alpert's and Scudamore's conviction that their healthy lifestyle is tied into their business success is a theme that was echoed by the more than two dozen entrepreneurs I interviewed for this book. These business owners come from a variety of backgrounds—some are lifelong entrepreneurs, while others discovered their passion after a corporate career. Some lead large companies, others have small businesses or solo concerns. Products range from high-tech medical devices to pet food to internet marketing. All of these entrepreneurs have their own motivations for working out and eating well, but the one thing they have in common is the firm belief that taking care of their health means they're taking care of their business.

In the pages that follow, these trailblazing company leaders give their tips and insights on how an entrepreneur can fit in exercise and good nutrition even with a hectic schedule (and offer some wisdom on business success along the way). You'll find practical techniques, simple solutions, and inspiring stories to help you live a healthier life, keeping in mind the unique demands you face in managing your time and energy.

Each chapter begins with a One-Minute Summary that hits the chapter's highlights and ends with Action Items—these boil the chapter down to a few specific steps that will help you quickly implement the chapter's concepts, usually with near-term deadlines to keep you on track. This book's purpose is to help you get fit, eat well, and stay healthy, but it should not take the place of your doctor's advice. Also, you should get medical clearance before embarking on a new nutrition or exercise program.

As an entrepreneur, you believe in action, and your motivation comes from deep within. You seize opportunity before it knocks and pursue your ambitions in the face of adversity. You marshal assets and convince others to believe in your vision, all the while adjusting course when a fast-changing world demands it. It's no wonder the English word entrepreneur traces its origin to the French word *entreprendre*—meaning "to undertake." In that spirit, this book is offered as a call to action to create a new vision, this one for yourself. My aim is to inspire you to undertake an active lifestyle, eat a well-balanced diet, and manage your stress. And in so doing, as Alpert and Scudamore and so many other thriving entrepreneurs have discovered, you'll see that your health is not only an important pursuit in itself—it's also integral to the success of your business.

*To my wife, Adrienne, and my parents, Robert and Vivian, for showing me what it means to follow your passion*

PART I

# *Healthy Due Diligence*

# CHAPTER 1

# The Fit Entrepreneur

> *If I'm healthy, then the company's going to be healthy . . .*
> *There's a direct correlation.*
>
> —DAN SANTY, SANTY ADVERTISING

---

**ONE-MINUTE SUMMARY**

- Research shows a connection between fitness and entrepreneurial success.
- Exercise and good nutrition boost brain function, creativity, self-confidence, and mood, as well as reduce anxiety, depression, and sick time—ensuring that you'll be there for your business on a day-to-day basis and for the long haul.
- Each of us is given a "stock of health"—if we spend it wisely by eating well and exercising, we will enjoy better quality of life in later years.
- Beginning a nutrition and exercise program is like launching a business—the odds are tough, but by tackling both with enthusiasm you will succeed.

Starting a business is one of the boldest moves you can make. It is a leap of faith—faith in yourself, your ideas, your intelligence, your drive. It means long hours, stress, and sometimes, waking up in the middle of the night wondering how you're going to make it through the next day. It takes guts to believe that you can offer a superior product and a faster service, that you have a unique vision of how things should be done.

As a result of your passion, you pour all you've got into making your ideas a reality. You study what your competitors are doing, where your industry is heading, and when to make your next innovation, all while keeping customers happy. You live a day with 24 hours, but you need 30.

So really, you don't have time for exercising and eating well. In a long list of things you need to accomplish, these are luxuries that you can afford to skip for the sake of your business, not to mention your personal and family life. It's better to send out that one last letter, phone the client you should have called two hours ago, or check the status of that shipment to Chicago. It's really, you might say, a good business decision to forgo the gym or to eat whatever's handy, whether it's a fast-food burger or a day-old sandwich out of a vending machine.

But wait a minute. As with any business decision, you need a closer look at how your lifestyle affects not only your health but also your bottom line. What you'll find when doing your due diligence—and what this book is about—is that eating right and exercising are two of the smartest things you can do for your business.

## THE BUSINESS-FITNESS CONNECTION

The truth is, a link between work and well-being isn't breaking news. Researchers have looked at whether staying healthy and fit can help an employee's chances of succeeding in business.

- One study found that commercial real-estate stockbrokers who had a regular running routine earned slightly larger sales commissions than nonrunning brokers. In a later study, researchers had employees from a hospital equipment company exercise 30 to 45 minutes a day at least four times per week. The workers showed significant improvement in productivity and job satisfaction compared with those who didn't exercise.

- A 2005 British study surveyed 200 employees who often made exercise part of their workdays. A majority of the workers thought their time management skills, mental performance, and potential to satisfy deadlines improved on the days they worked out.

Similarly, larger companies are seeing the benefits of healthy employees and setting up employee wellness programs. For example, General Motors reportedly has saved nearly $5 for every dollar spent on its wellness program (see the sidebar "A Weighty Cost to Business"). But until recently, not much attention has been paid to how a healthy lifestyle affects entrepreneurial success. That is, until a group of business school professors who specialize in entrepreneurship noticed that many successful entrepreneurs also were in good shape.

## LOOKING AT ENTREPRENEURS

To test the idea that regular physical activity translated to the business owner's bottom line, Michael G. Goldsby, Ph.D., of Ball State University in Muncie, Indiana, and his colleagues surveyed 366 small businesspeople in the Midwest to determine if they ran or lifted weights and, if so, how that affected their business and their psychological outlook.

Goldsby and his colleagues began by identifying a key difference between the typical corporate employee and the entrepreneur: The corporate employee can often afford more time to go work out—maybe even at the company gym. "The business is still going to run," explains Goldsby, the Stoops Distinguished Professor of Entrepreneurship in Ball State's Department of Marketing and Management, Miller College of Business (www.bsu.edu/entrepreneurship). By comparison, "entrepreneurs are the face of the company," he says. "So we wanted to find out if time spent away from the business working out was time well spent. And what we found was, it is."

Entrepreneurs who take a brief absence from the business—for example, to go jogging at lunch—do not leave a void that hurts the business, even if one or just a handful of people are running the whole show. In fact, Goldsby and his colleagues discovered that entrepreneurs who ran enjoyed better sales than nonrunners. What's more, those who ran or lifted weights scored higher in measures of personal satisfaction, independence, and autonomy. "Our research showed that for an entrepreneur," Goldsby says, "exercise is a good investment."

And anecdotal evidence backs up the research. Numerous entrepreneurs who contributed their insights to this book confirmed that their businesses benefit from adopting a healthy lifestyle. "I used to think that I couldn't make the time to work out and eat well," says Brian Scudamore, founder and CEO of 1-800-GOT-JUNK? "Now I realize I can't afford not to make the time."

Entrepreneur Max Hoes agrees. He's the co-owner of CFR Line, an international transportation company specializing in ocean export of automobiles. "It's a very simple business, but it's very hectic, with a million things to do a day," he says. "Exercise keeps me calm and my stress level low. It helps me in solving problems, and despite the time working out takes, it makes it easier to manage my day. It seems like sometimes when you do more, it's easy to get more done."

## A WEIGHTY COST TO BUSINESS

A two-year study published in 2003 in the *American Journal of Health Promotion* found that obese workers at General Motors (GM) experienced up to $1,500 more in yearly medical costs than employees with a healthy weight. When you consider that more than 20 percent of the GM workers fell under the category of obese, the impact of those costs becomes staggering.

Almost 90 percent of small businesses reported paying more to provide medical insurance for their workers in 2005 compared with 2004. Half the companies surveyed indicated year-over-year jumps of between 10 and 20 percent. About 10 percent reported increases of 30 percent or more.

Therefore, it's no surprise that a number of larger companies are installing health-promotion and disease-prevention programs for their workers. In fact, some of these programs actually started decades ago. The returns on investment have been impressive. In a recent review of nine big employers, for each dollar spent on a health program, they saved between $1.49 and $4.91—with GM obtaining the high end. For tips on starting your own workplace wellness program, see Appendix A.

Let's look at why spending some time away from the business to boost health actually boosts the bottom line.

### Building a Habit of Persistence

Entrepreneurship isn't always easy, and neither is eating well or exercising. If they were, we'd have many more entrepreneurs and a lot more fit people around. But here's the other side of the coin: building a habit of exercise and good nutrition can translate to how you run your company. "The focus that you get," Goldsby says, "carries over into other aspects of your life because you gain perseverance, self discipline, and I think to a great degree, self confidence." Robert Smith, who founded and runs Robert Smith & Associates Public Relations, agrees. "The same mental toughness of working out applies to business," he says. "I call it the killer instinct."

### Keeping You In the Game

Illness can result in long-term disruptive absences. In fact, when an entrepreneur becomes synonymous with the identity of the business, his sickness or death could spell the death of the company. This is an important correlation, considering that research on entrepreneurs indicates that there are lots of cases of bad backs, digestion problems, insomnia, or headaches.

Exercise and eating well not only help keep you healthy so you can be there for your business, they build the endurance needed for the daily demands you face. Dan Santy, who founded and operates Santy Advertising, watches his nutrition and keeps active by hiking, doing indoor cycling classes, and working out with a personal trainer three days a week. "I bet you I'm sick one day a year, if that," Santy says. "Especially when the flu season comes along, I just never seem to get hit by it."

> *I find that the more I work out, the less tired I am, oddly enough.*
>
> —Dominic Rubino, president of Fulcrum Agency, a business consulting firm

### Providing a Sounding Board

Entrepreneurs often live a lonely business life. They may be in contact with customers, employees, and attorneys, but they may not have someone else who can act as a confidant for discussing new ideas, employee

## FARM-RAISED FITNESS

Richard Thompson has been an entrepreneur since his high school days, when he started a business that he later sold to Pizza Hut. He's founded multiple companies, including the American Italian Pasta Company. Trading people food for cat cuisine, he is now CEO and "Top Cat" of The Meow Mix Company.

Having grown up on a farm, he prefers early morning workouts such as a ten-mile bike ride, a three-mile run, or a gym session. After his runs and rides, he says, he always has new thoughts about the business to write down and take to work. "When you have a bunch of ideas and you're ready to talk to people," he adds, "you energize the office, and it sets a whole different tone."

In the winter, skiing provides another outlet for staying active and relieving stress. "As you're going down that hill, you're not thinking about anything other than getting to the bottom." Still, at age 54, Thompson says it takes diligence to stick to his healthy lifestyle. "I've noticed in the last couple of years that I really have to exercise and watch what I eat," he says. "You have to continue doing something with your body every day."

issues, or that difficult client. Entrepreneurs also are so buried in their business that they may lack a social outlet. Having workout buddies gives a business owner a group of friends outside of the business and a support group that could act as a good sounding board if one isn't available at the office.

### *Boosting Brain Function*

Breakthroughs in neuroscience since the late 1990s have given insights into how physical activity may affect the brain. Research is showing that exercise benefits the hippocampus, a part of the brain that is a key to memory and learning. In fact, scientists are now refuting the conventional wisdom that the brain stops producing new cells after childhood—finding that it actually keeps creating cells throughout life. A 1999 study published in the journal *Nature Neuroscience* revealed that adult mice who had access to running wheels saw a two-fold increase in the amount of new brain cells formed in the hippocampus. Also, animal studies are establishing that exercise helps protect the brain from stress and infection.

### *Maintaining Your Sharpness*

Similar to exercise, a nutritious diet also can boost brain power. There is evidence to suggest that saturated fat can harm the brain, while fruits and vegetables such as strawberries, blueberries, and spinach can have a positive impact. Aging rats that ate a diet of these foods for two months had improved brain cell function and did better on a memory test when compared with rats on a normal diet. In other research, rats fed a diet with 40 percent of calories from saturated fat faired poorly on memory and learning tests. If rodents don't convince you, then there's this: a study published in the journal *Archives of Neurology* in 2003 looked at more than 800 people and found that those folks who ate the most saturated fat had more than double the risk of Alzheimer's disease compared to those people who ate the least.

Think about it this way: food, just like a drug your doctor might prescribe, can alter the chemical stew of your brain—the effect just may not be as pronounced, so we tend not to make that connection. Of course, to understand this brain-stomach connection all you have to do is think about the times you've been too wired to

---

## WHAT'S THE NET WORTH OF FITNESS?

Staying fit and maintaining a healthy weight may have a direct association with people's financial situations as they age, at least for women. Researchers analyzed 1998 data on more than 7,000 men and women from the University of Michigan Health and Retirement Study and found that the weight of middle-aged women had a correlation to their net worth.

A woman who was moderately to severely obese and between 57 and 67 years old had a net worth about 60 percent less than that of her nonobese female peer. On average, that translated to a difference of around $135,670. (Obesity's connection to the bank accounts of men were smaller and not statistically significant.)

---

sleep because you had coffee late at night or when you've eaten the spaghetti special for lunch and felt like taking a nap an hour later.

"Our mental function is directly related to what we eat or don't eat," write Arthur Winter, M.D., and Ruth Winter, M.S., in *Smart Food: Diet and Nutrition for Maximum Brain Power* (St. Martin's Press, 1999). Food, they explain, ultimately becomes the chemicals in the brain that affect mood, memory, appetite, even intelligence.

## Cultivating Creativity

Physical movement may be a key to overcoming creativity "blocks." In a study published in 1997 in the *British Journal of Sports Medicine*, researchers reported that people who participated in an aerobic workout or aerobic dance significantly boosted their creativity compared with their results after simply watching a video. Not surprisingly, the subjects also saw an increase in positive mood after exercise and a significant drop in positive mood after watching the video.

Professor Goldsby, who conducted the entrepreneur-fitness study, is now looking into the ties between exercise and entrepreneurial creativity, and says he expects to find a link. "My belief," says Goldsby, who is an avid long-distance runner, "is that some of your best ideas will come when you're working out, when you least expect it." When it comes to ideas, he explains, the brain does two things—it creates the ideas and then evaluates them. But the evaluation can happen almost immediately, and this can hinder the entire creative process. "You've got to really turn off your judgmental side to let ideas develop," he says. "A lot of people in their daily routines at work are in that judgmental, critical mode."

This is where exercise comes in: It can offer a break from the workplace that gives your subconscious a chance to foster ideas and lets you drop the "veil of critical thinking" that can disrupt the creative process, Goldsby says. Jogging, for example, can be a meditative-like pursuit, as you get lost in the calming sound of your own breathing. "When we're in that moment, our judgment drops, and that allows ideas to come forth that would not come forth when you're in your daily routine of work," Goldsby says. "One of the best things about doing your exercise is a chance to get in an almost Zen state, and let ideas form."

Again, anecdotal evidence reveals that active entrepreneurs find some of their best ideas come not while sitting behind a desk, but while being physical. For Jennifer Melton—who with her husband founded Cloud Star, a pet food company specializing in natural products—most of her business concepts materialize while hiking. Away from phones, e-mail, and countless other interruptions, creativity is free to blossom into an "I've got it" moment. "You're walking along talking and just enjoying being outside, and something will come to you," she says. "I would say that nine out of ten of our ideas come to us while we're hiking."

### Maintaining Mental Health

Anxiety is a business owner's constant companion—especially in the start-up phase of a company. But here, too, being active can play a positive role. Exercise can improve mood and help out when you feel depressed or anxious. Moving your body increases the levels of mood-boosting neurotransmitters and endorphins in your brain, reduces muscle tension, improves sleep, and cuts down levels of cortisol (a stress hormone). Basically, physical activity serves as your own personal pressure-relief valve, allowing your brain to take a break from the daily routine. In practical terms, it's nearly impossible to feel nervous, angry, or frustrated *and* be breaking a sweat at the same time.

Mentally, exercise has numerous benefits, according to Mayo Clinic psychologist Kristin Vickers-Douglas, Ph.D. These include distraction from negative thoughts, improved self-confidence, and a sense of accomplishment from achieving a goal. These are especially important for an entrepreneur: projecting a sense of assurance will help you gain the trust of your clients.

But even more importantly, you don't always have control over your business—i.e., fickle customers, tardy suppliers, capricious employees—but each and every day you have absolute control over your exercise and nutrition. At the end of the day, no matter what else went right or wrong, if you did something active and made a few smart food choices, you can pat yourself on the back for a job well done.

## IT'S YOUR HEALTH CAPITAL—SPEND IT WISELY

While there are immediate payoffs for you and your business in adopting a healthy lifestyle, not all the benefits are so near term. The choices you make today could affect your quality of life in the years to come—say, in your retirement years when you'd like to enjoy the fruits of your hard work. In a study published in the *Journal of the American Medical Association* in 2003, researchers estimated that the years of life lost due to severe obesity ranged from 5 to 20, depending on gender and race. And that tells only part of the story; excess weight also can affect the number of disability-free years a person enjoys. When you take into account physical quality of life, the effects of obesity are actually equivalent to 30 years of aging, according to research published in 2002 in the journal *Health Affairs*.

You can think about healthy living in economic terms. Health economists—yes, there are such experts—say each of us is "endowed with a certain stock of

---

## THE HEALTH CONSEQUENCES

According to a 2003 report issued by the U.S. Department of Health and Human Services, being overweight or obese raises the risk for a number of conditions:

- Type 2 diabetes
- High blood pressure
- High cholesterol levels
- Coronary heart disease
- Congestive heart failure
- Angina pectoris
- Stroke
- Asthma
- Osteoarthritis
- Musculoskeletal disorders

- Gallbladder disease
- Sleep apnea and respiratory issues
- Gout
- Bladder control difficulties
- Poor reproductive health for women, including pregnancy complications, menstrual abnormalities, infertility, and irregular ovulation

- Cancers of the uterus, breast, prostate, kidney, liver, pancreas, esophagus, colon, and rectum

---

health," and this stock either helps or hinders how much satisfaction we achieve over the course of our lives. As researchers in one academic article put it, "A fit 65-year-old retiree may be able to travel, dance, or ski, while another 65-year-old is unable to walk long distances or to live without medication."

Ultimately, according to the economic theory, we weigh the hassles of leading a healthy life today—comparing nutrition labels, for example—with our perceived payoff in the future. If we don't put much value on our quality of life in the future—or simply don't give it much thought—then we're less likely to do much about exercise and eating well now. Think about your own "economic" model and whether you're discounting the future value of your health as you age in order to avoid perceived short-term inconveniences of activity and good nutrition.

## THE BUSINESS OF FITNESS

In taking on the life of an entrepreneur, of course, you've had to overcome difficult odds. No one gives you a guarantee that your business will be successful. Instead, you do your best to know what you're getting into and then take a plunge into the unknown. And every day you roll up your sleeves, face down the odds, and dig in.

This is the mindset you'll need for a healthy lifestyle. Going for a walk takes effort, and only you will make the decision to eat more whole grains, fruits, and veggies. The odds of success seem long. Fewer than one-third of adults in the United States are physically active on a regular basis. Research has found that even among adults trying to lose or maintain their weight, fewer than 20 percent were complying with guidelines on boosting physical activity and cutting calories. But taking on challenges is what you do, and this is no different.

> *I train every day, either in the gym or biking or running out on the road. I've found that exercise provides a really good balance for business activities because it takes all of that daily stress out of your system, calming you down. And also, when you're training a lot, it allows you to do some really good, solid thinking. You get into a zone, and when you're in that zone, things seem a little clearer.*
>
> —Stanley Wunderlich, chairman and CEO of Consulting for Strategic Growth 1 Ltd., a Wall Street investor-relations company

## A LITTLE GOES A LONG WAY

When it comes to weight control and health, small changes make a big difference. You simply need to make incremental steps away from the direction you've been heading and toward a new path—however small those steps may be at first. Realize this:

- Losing between 5 to 15 percent of excess weight can cut the risk for some chronic disorders.

- A 10 percent reduction in cholesterol levels may decrease the incidence of heart disease by 30 percent.

- One year after quitting smoking, the extra risk of heart disease from a nicotine habit is cut by half. After 15 years without a cigarette, the risk is the same as it would be for someone who never smoked.

So as with your business, starting your fitness and nutrition program won't be a cakewalk. This book isn't about effortless workouts and eating all the high-fat bacon you want. It's about developing a healthy mindset that will last a lifetime. In the chapters ahead, you'll be given easy-to-implement fitness and nutrition tools to do just that. But you must tackle this part of your life with the enthusiasm you have for your business. If you do, you will succeed.

The great news is that it will get easier as you go, as you form the habits of your new healthier lifestyle. To paraphrase Newton's first law of motion, a body at rest will stay at rest, and a body in motion will keep going unless some outside force tries to stop it. With fitness and nutrition, that same law applies. Stay at rest, and it's tough to get moving. But once you get the motion started, it becomes increasingly difficult to stop.

Once you take the stairs a couple times a week instead of the elevator, once you pack an apple for an afternoon snack three days in a row, you've started instilling a powerful pattern in your life. You'll see that in just a short time, these actions can snowball and take on a momentum that will be unstoppable. As Mark

Andrus, co-founder of Stacy's Pita Chip Company, says: "Exercise has just become such a part of my lifestyle and a part of my everyday schedule, and I really look forward to it. Work can be stressful, but then I can go to the gym or go for a run and I feel better and ready for the next day."

◆ ◆ ◆ ◆ ◆

## THE BOTTOM LINE

You've picked up the book, you've taken action. Go a little further. Take the next step and turn the page. You'll find a quick start to a healthier, more vigorous life, with advice and words of encouragement from your fellow entrepreneurs who've made fitness and good nutrition part of their lifestyle.

---

### *Action* Item

➤ Take a minute to reflect on how your health and fitness may have affected your business in the past year.

---

# CHAPTER 2

# The Quick-Start Action Plan

*Just get busy doing something . . . My advice is to start small.*

—ROBERT SMITH, FOUNDER AND PRESIDENT OF

ROBERT SMITH & ASSOCIATES PUBLIC RELATIONS

## ONE-MINUTE SUMMARY

- In adopting a healthy lifestyle, start small and build on your successes.
- The Quick-Start Action Plan gives you three targets this week.

    1. Exercise at your desk.

    2. Take ten-minute energy walks.

    3. Drink ice water and save five bites from one daily meal.

- As you adopt more advanced exercises, you can use the Quick-Start Action Plan exercises to take de-stress breaks during the day or when you're too short on time for longer exercise sessions.

Taking the first steps in something new can be daunting. But almost *any* action—no matter how small—puts momentum on your side.

While each entrepreneur has a different path to success, everyone starts with that first step forward; you must take action, even without being entirely sure of the outcome. Those who hesitate to take that step, to turn idea into deed, are forever stuck with the status quo—not risking failure but also not finding fortune.

> *In starting a business, I think you should try things you believe in. Of course, you need to have some confidence, but you need to try your idea and not be afraid. I think the biggest thing that holds people back is the fear they may fail. Don't be afraid of failure.*
>
> —MAX HOES, CO-OWNER OF AUTOMOBILE EXPORT COMPANY CFR LINE

This chapter is about the first step, about taking action right now, for your health and fitness. This three-prong Quick-Start Action Plan targets your muscles, your heart, and your nutrition. The plan is based on the same guiding principle that can build a solid company. "Start with limited capital so you don't stress the heck out of yourself," says 1-800-GOT-JUNK? founder and CEO Brian Scudamore. "I started with a thousand bucks, and if I lost my thousand dollars, it wasn't the end of the world . . . Start small, build the business up over time, and have patience."

That's exactly the secret to eating well and getting fit—start small and build on your successes. So now is the moment to institute healthy habits into your daily routine, easily and in a way that's time efficient. It just takes *starting*.

## QUICK-START EXERCISE

At its most basic level, exercise is nothing more than your muscles, bones, and heart working as they were designed so well to do—to move. And even with a crowded schedule, you can work physical activity into your life just about anywhere and with minimal equipment.

If you're at the office, take a 15-minute break in the morning or afternoon to complete this session—and you'll have your first workout under your belt before you go home. If you're at home, take 15 minutes before lunch or dinner to knock out the routine. The movements are unobtrusive—you can think of them as "stealth" exercises.

This first step will serve as a springboard to more fitness and dietary changes in your life. And once you learn these movements, the more challenging habit changes will be easier. But even when you become more advanced, or if you are right now, these simple exercises provide a refreshing break during the day. They can also serve as a fast workout for those inevitable times when your schedule is too hectic for longer workouts.

Still, if you do nothing with this book other than take away these exercises and this chapter's action plan, you'll be doing something powerful for your body and mind.

A note on terminology: A "repetition" or "rep" is one complete movement of a given exercise. A "set" is a given number repetitions done in sequence. Start by doing one set for each exercise—if you feel good, you can add a second set. Do two sessions this week.

### Desk Exercises

CHAIR LEG EXTENSION

*Muscles strengthened*: Quadriceps (thighs)

Press your tailbone firmly against the back of the chair. If the chair is adjustable, move the height so your thighs are parallel to the ground. Lightly grasp the armrests or the edges of the seat pad. Keeping your back straight and looking straight ahead, slowly extend your right leg with your foot flexed toward your shin. At the top of the movement, your leg should be fully extended, but don't forcefully lock out your knee. Slowly return to the starting position. Do 10 repetitions, then repeat with your left leg (this is one set).

ISOMETRIC HAND PRESS

*Muscles strengthened*: Biceps, triceps, chest

Sitting upright in your chair, grasp your hands together in front of your chest, and firmly press them together. Make sure you continue to breathe throughout the exercise. Hold for 10 seconds and then relax for 10 seconds, then repeat four more times.

WALL PUSH-OFF

*Muscles strengthened*: Chest, triceps, shoulders

Stand about three feet from a wall, and place your hands flush against the wall, about shoulder-width apart. Slowly lower your body toward the wall by flexing your elbows. When your elbows are aligned with your torso, push back up. Do 10 repetitions. Make this exercise more challenging by using your desk: Stand several feet away and position your hands on the edge of the desk, shoulder-width apart. Then repeat the raising and lowering of your body by flexing your elbows.

### Overhead Press

*Muscles strengthened*: Shoulders

Sitting upright in your chair, flex your elbows so that your left hand is in front of your left shoulder, and your right hand is in front of your right shoulder. Your elbows should be slightly flared out to the sides, just below shoulder-level. Lightly clench your fists with palms facing forward. Next, fully extend your elbows without locking them out, with your hands moving toward the center

---

## FORM CHECK

When doing these exercises and stretches, keep these tips in mind:

- *Don't hold your breath.* Keep breathing normally during each exercise; holding your breath can spike your blood pressure.

- *Keep your spine in its "neutral position."* To find this position, lie on your back and arch your lower back (this is called extension). Then round the lower back (flexion). The neutral position is midway between these extremes.

- *Move in a slow and controlled manner.* This will help avoid injury and maintain good tension in your muscles.

- *Hold stretches for 15 to 30 seconds.* This will allow your muscles to adjust to the increased range of motion.

- *Don't bounce.* This could cause a muscle to spontaneously tighten because its defense mechanism is trying to protect it from overstretching. Not only does this defeat the purpose of stretching, but it could cause a strain.

over your head. Slowly return to the starting position. Complete 10 reps. To make the exercise more difficult, use a book to press overhead.

DRAWING-IN MANEUVER

*Muscles strengthened*: Mid-section

Sit upright on the edge of your chair, grasping the arm rests or the edges of the seat pad. You can also stand with your hands on your hips, feet shoulder-width apart. Next, pull your stomach up and in as far as possible—think of pulling your belly button toward your spine. Hold that position for the count of five to ten, then release. Do 5 to 8 repetitions.

## Flexibility Exercises

SIDE BEND

*Muscles stretched*: Back and sides

Sit at the edge of your chair with your back straight, and interlace your fingers with your palms facing away from you. Reach your arms straight above your head, then lean to the left from the waist and hold. Next lean to the right and hold.

CROSS ARM

*Muscles stretched*: Upper back

Sit upright and bring your right arm across your upper body at about shoulder level. Your elbow should be slightly flexed. With your left hand, grasp under your right arm just above the elbow. Gently pull your right arm across your chest, toward the left, and hold. Don't shrug your shoulders—keep them relaxed. Repeat with your left arm across your upper body.

NECK STRETCH

*Muscles stretched*: Neck

Sit or stand with your head upright. Slowly turn your head to the right as far as comfortably possible and hold, then turn slowly to the left and hold. Next, let your head fall gently toward your chest and hold. Avoid tilting your head backward—it weighs about 10 pounds, so this can put too much stress on your upper spine.

## WORKOUT BOX

| Desk Exercise | Repetitions | Sets |
|---|---|---|
| Chair leg extension | 10 each side | 1–2 |
| Isometric hand press | 5 | 1–2 |
| Wall push-off | 10 | 1–2 |
| Overhead press | 10 | 1–2 |
| Drawing-in maneuver | 5–8 | 1–2 |

| Flexibility Exercise | Repetitions | Sets |
|---|---|---|
| Side bend | 1 | 1 |
| Cross arm | 1 | 1 |
| Neck stretch | 1 | 1 |

## QUICK-START CARDIO—THE TEN-MINUTE ENERGY WALK

An energy walk is a faster-paced walk done with an exaggerated arm swing. You'll eventually go for longer walks—and possibly jogs (see Chapter 9)—but for now the aim is to get moving, and there's no better way to do that than going for a walk. Why walk? Because walking raises your heart rate, which burns calories and makes your cardiovascular system stronger, and it tones your leg muscles. It's also a wonderful stress reliever. "I still walk to and from work once or twice a week," says entrepreneur Brian Scudamore. "It's a great unwinding mechanism."

Plus, there's no learning curve, and it's low-impact, so there is minimal stress to your joints. You can walk alone to enjoy the solitude of your own thoughts or go with business partners, employees, and friends for some social time or to brainstorm issues at work. Or maybe invite along a client—exercise can be a great bonding experience. Walking also doesn't require much special equipment or clothing—although you should wear shoes with thick flexible soles to provide a cushion for your feet (consider investing in a comfortable pair of walking or running shoes, for around $70).

Aim to walk three times this week. Before you head out the door, keep these tips in mind:

- Use the first two or three minutes to warm up at a slow pace, then increase your speed to a pace that feels brisk—but you should still be able to carry on a conversation.
- To maintain good posture, look straight ahead and keep your back straight.
- Your hands should be in a relaxed, cupped position, and your elbows constantly flexed to about 90 degrees.
- Allow your hands to swing up to about chest level, but don't let your arms flare out from the sides of your body.
- Keep a slight flex in your knees—locking out can cause injury.

## FOUNDING FATHERS OF ENERGY WALKS

If founding a country holds lessons for entrepreneurs starting companies, John Adams and Thomas Jefferson have something to teach. Adams took walks between five to ten miles to "rouse the spirits," according to David McCullough's biography of the second president. During his time in Paris, after breakfast Adams and his son (future president John Quincy) typically "set off for a five- or six-mile walk . . . before getting down to work."

In a letter to a student in August 1785, Jefferson said that "walking is the best possible exercise. Habituate yourself to walk very far." He advised that "health must not be sacrificed to learning. A strong body makes a mind strong . . . . The object of walking is to relax the mind. You should therefore not permit yourself even to think while you walk; but divert your attention by the objects surrounding you."

## THE BEST TIME TO EXERCISE

What time of day should you work out? In general, the body performs best and has the least risk of injuries in late afternoon and early evening, according to *The Body Clock Guide to Better Health* (Henry Holt and Company, 2000) by Michael Smolensky, Ph.D., and Lynne Lamberg. A workout around that time also may help promote sleep later. On the other hand, exercising outside during daytime exposes you to bright light and helps maintain proper body rhythms. With all that said, the best time to exercise is when it makes sense in your schedule and when you feel like you have the most energy.

- Strike the ground with heels first, toes pointed straight ahead.
- Wear sunscreen.
- If you make an appointment to walk with someone else, you'll be much more likely to make the scheduled time.

## QUICK-START NUTRITION

To get a quick start on eating healthier, two simple adjustments to your daily routine are all that's required right now. You'll get a more comprehensive dietary plan in Chapter 7—and even then you won't be counting calories or making complicated meals—but these changes will immediately make a difference in your nutrition.

### Drink Ice Water with Meals and When Thirsty During the Day

Your body will warm the water, and this will require a caloric expenditure. In fact, when compared with drinking water at room temperature, consuming eight ounces of ice water can expend about 9 extra calories. Doesn't sound like much? If you do that three times a day, it adds up to nearly 10,000 calories in a year—that's almost three pounds with virtually no effort.

Beyond the calorie-burning benefits, making water a habit makes sense. Water helps foods break down to their basic elements; provides a cushion for your body's organs, including the brain; and regulates your temperature through perspiration. Water makes up between 45 to 70 percent of body weight, and is the most plentiful chemical material in your body. For purposes of controlling or losing weight, some research indicates that water can promote a feeling of fullness when it's consumed with a meal or incorporated into food.

For Jennifer Melton, co-founder of Cloud Star natural pet products, water is an integral part of her workday. "I always keep a glass of water at my desk," she says. "It gives me energy and sustains my energy throughout the day. When I start dragging, sometimes the easiest thing to do is drink a glass of water."

### *Save Five Bites*

Portion sizes in recent decades have greatly expanded. Offerings in fast-food restaurants, for example, can be between two and five times the original size. In the 1950s, a Burger King hamburger weighed 3.9 ounces, but now you can order a Double Whopper at a hefty 12.6 ounces. Restaurants use bigger plates, and pizza is made in larger pans. Even frozen diet meals from Lean Cuisine and Weight Watchers have touted larger package sizes. These larger portions pack more calories and prompt you to eat too much. A small size of McDonald's french fries sports 210 calories, while the supersize version contains 610 calories. Given that Americans spend

---

### HOW MUCH $H_2O$?

Maybe you've heard the common advice to drink eight 8-ounce glasses of water a day, and that coffee, tea, and soft drinks don't count because caffeinated drinks dehydrate you. It's not clear where this "rule" came from, but there doesn't appear to be scientific evidence to back it up.

A 2004 report from the Institute of Medicine of the National Academies gives a general daily guideline of 91 ounces of water for women and 125 ounces for men—but that's counting total water from all beverages and foods (about 20 percent of water intake comes from food). Most healthy people actually meet their daily hydration needs by letting thirst be their guide, according to the report.

---

## A DOG'S TALE

One of the ways business founder and executive Jennifer Melton stays in shape is to run with her dog Samantha. "Dogs make great workout partners because they're enthusiastic and they love exercise," Melton says. "Samantha has definitely helped me keep up my running routine and healthy lifestyle." But her four-legged friend is more than a faithful workout companion—Samantha also provided the spark that launched Melton's entrepreneurial success.

In 1998, Melton and Brennan Johnson adopted Samantha as a puppy from a local animal shelter. The couple quickly learned that the German shepherd mix had food allergies and a sensitive stomach. Unable to find a diet that would agree with the pup, Melton and Johnson began baking wholesome treats for Samantha. They then contributed some of those treats to a local bake sale at the San Clemente Animal Shelter. "The reception was overwhelming," Johnson says. Soon people were calling asking about the goodies, and that was enough for the couple to take $20,000 in personal savings plus Small Business Administration financing and launch Cloud Star, dedicated to bringing pets wholesome and tasty food. Melton left a job working for a clothing company, Johnson quit his career as a structural engineer, and they haven't looked back.

Now they go to work every day with Samantha and another adopted dog, Nala. "I'm living my dream," Melton says. "I get up every morning invigorated to start my day."

Growing up in entrepreneurial families, Melton and Johnson knew firsthand the stresses of a small business and the lack of a regular paycheck. But they also saw the excitement and challenge that make entrepreneurship so rewarding. Still, Melton says, when considering a business, it's important to find something that you love. "It has to be passion driven," she says. "Or else I think it would just get really tiring, really quickly. You can run on excitement and adrenalin for a year or two, and after that you have to love what you do. You know, life is so short to hate going to work every day."

nearly 50 percent of their food dollars outside the home, it makes sense that by the mid-1990s people were eating 200 more calories per day compared with the late 1970s.

One reason behind the trend is that price competition has caused manufacturers to offer larger items. Also, restaurant owners say it comes down to value—customers want more food for their dollar. Whatever the reason, it's clear that we're getting more food placed in front of us than we used to, and that leads to excessive eating.

Here's what to do: to help control your portions, at one meal during the day, simply save five bites of your food. You can mentally account for the bites, or you can actually partition them off to the side. Do this whether it's a restaurant, fast-food, or home-cooked meal. If you think this sounds trivial, consider this: If the average meal has 350 calories and you usually take 20 bites per meal, you'll save about 90 calories per day or 32,000 calories per year—*which equates to more than nine pounds a year.*

If you're in a restaurant and it's convenient, ask for a doggy bag before you begin your meal—set the five bites aside. You can snack on them later in the day (make sure to refrigerate, if necessary). The point is to reduce the portion size of the food that's in front of you, right now.

As you get comfortable with these changes in lifestyle—adding movement to your day with exercises and walking, and starting to gain control over your eating habits—you'll enjoy the powerful feeling that positive change can bring to your life and your business.

---

### *Action* Item

➤ As you successfully complete each element of the Quick-Start Action Plan in the following week, check off the boxes below.

---

## THE QUICK-START ACTION PLAN

**Desk Exercises (twice this week)**

_____    _____ Chair leg extension

_____    _____ Isometric hand press

_____    _____ Wall push-off

_____    _____ Overhead press

_____    _____ Drawing-in maneuver

**Flexibility Exercises (twice this week)**

_____    _____ Side bend

_____    _____ Cross arm

_____    _____ Neck stretch

**The Ten-Minute Energy Walk (three times this week)**

____    ____    ____

**Nutrition (every day this week)**

*Glass of ice water with meals and when thirsty*

____    ____    ____    ____    ____    ____    ____

*Saving five bites (at one meal every day this week)*

____    ____    ____    ____    ____    ____    ____

# CHAPTER 3

# Myth Busting

*The biggest mistake people make is that they do too much too soon. With lifting weights and working out, you always want to err on the conservative side. So if you think you can do a dumbbell curl exercise with 25 pounds, for example, do it with 15 pounds instead. Start off very, very conservatively.*

—MARK PLAATJES, PHYSICAL THERAPIST AND CO-FOUNDER OF BOULDER RUNNING COMPANY, A MULTILOCATION RUNNING STORE IN COLORADO

**ONE-MINUTE SUMMARY**

- 🕐 Fitness and nutrition myths are common—don't let these be a barrier to your getting fit.
- 🕐 Some of the common misconceptions (and their corresponding realities) covered in this chapter include:
  - *It's too late for me to exercise.* Ninety-year olds can build muscle.
  - *A woman will get too bulky if she lifts weights.* It's unlikely because she lacks sufficient testosterone.

- *It takes too much time to eat right and exercise.* You can accumulate short bouts of activity throughout the day, and even just ten minutes of exercise can boost your mood and energy.
- *I won't be able to enjoy my favorite foods.* Indulging occasionally is fine, and an "all-or-nothing" attitude is a recipe for failure.
- *No pain, no gain.* Exercise doesn't have to be painful; a brisk but comfortable walk can suffice.
- *It's inevitable that I'll gain weight as I age, so it's not worth fighting it.* Lifting weights adds muscle, which helps burn calories and along with aerobic exercise and eating wisely, combats middle-age spread.

Entrepreneurship is ripe ground for myth making. For example, to be successful, you have to be "born" an entrepreneur. That is unless, of course, you get lucky enough to be one of those "overnight" successes. Or, just possibly, you may strike gold by discovering the secret to "getting rich quick." These kinds of fictions are convenient ways to explain the rising and falling fortunes of the world of business, and they're harmless—except if you buy into them. Then they can become excuses for throwing in the towel on your business ambitions or, worse, not even trying in the first place.

For the same reason, you need to dispel any erroneous ideas you may have about diet and exercise, and the barriers you think you'll face. In nutrition and fitness—as in business—good information is key, but misinformation and myths abound. So know the facts, and don't let these ten myths keep you from getting in shape.

## MYTH 1: I'M NOT ATHLETIC, SO EVEN IF I WANTED TO BECOME MORE ACTIVE, I CAN'T DO IT

***Reality Check:*** *There are many ways to incorporate more physical activity into your day*

Being active can take many forms and your body will burn calories with whatever type of movement you do.

Increasing activity throughout your day can include things you may not have thought of. Parking your car a few extra blocks from the office, taking the stairs in your building, standing up and pacing while on the phone, visiting your employee down the hall instead of sending an e-mail—these things take energy, and that means they eat up calories. Even when you fidget, you burn calories! In fact, in a 2005 study published in the journal *Science*, Mayo Clinic researchers looked at ten

---

### CRUNCHING CALORIES

The number of calories you burn when your body moves is affected by several things.

- The more muscle mass involved in your movement, the more calories you burn at any particular level of exertion. So jogging, for example, consumes more calories than riding a stationary bike because running requires upper-body movement.

- Because it takes more effort to move a larger mass, a heavier person expends more calories than a lighter person doing the same activity.

- Activities that are weight-bearing burn more calories than activities that provide some support in counteracting the effect of gravity. So, for example, running tends to be more calorie-intense than swimming—if you're giving it the same effort level.

- If you're really good at an activity, your body's movements are more efficient, and so you burn fewer calories. The upside is that you can keep up the activity for a longer period of time because you won't tire as quickly.

---

lean and ten obese individuals, and found that the obese subjects averaged two hours more of sitting per day than their slim counterparts. That resulted in *350 fewer calories burned.* "Calories that people burn in their everyday activities . . . are far, far more important in obesity than we previously imagined," said one of the scientists in a press release.

Household chores are another source of calorie burning—sweeping requires almost 300 calories an hour, while shoveling snow can melt nearly 500. You'll even keep burning calories *after* you complete an activity—generally, for every 100 calories expended while active, you'll burn about 15 calories afterward. For a comprehensive list of activities and the number of calories they burn, check out Appendix B.

The bottom line is, you don't have to have a great jump shot, run a seven-minute mile, or even be coordinated to get active. You just have to get your body moving.

## MYTH 2: IT'S TOO LATE FOR ME TO EXERCISE

*Reality Check: Research shows that even those in their 90s can build new muscle and improve their speed*

Maybe you haven't exercised since high school gym class or you've been away from activity since you've launched your business. You've spent too many late nights and eaten too many bacon ultimate cheeseburgers. Even if you had the time, it's too late to do anything about it now, right?

Wrong. In the January 2005 issue of the *Journal of Applied Physiology*, researchers Christian K. Roberts and R. James Barnard tackle this issue head on. "The evidence is overwhelming," they write, "that physical activity and diet can reduce the risk of developing numerous chronic diseases, including [coronary artery disease], hypertension, diabetes, metabolic syndrome, and several forms of cancer, and in many cases in fact reverse existing disease." And in a 1990 study conducted at the U. S. Department of Agriculture, Human Nutrition Research Center on Aging at Tufts University in Massachusetts, researchers looked at the effects of strength training on frail senior adults with an average age of 90. After eight weeks of high-intensity training, the participants averaged strength gains of 174 percent,

## YOUR MUSCLES OR YOUR LIFE

Researchers are finding that strength may help people live longer and that the greatest health boost comes when moving from low to moderate strength. One 25-year study categorized men based on grip strength. Those in the top three strongest groups, respectively, had a 49.1 percent, 34.4 percent, and 28.5 percent decreased risk of death compared with those in the weakest group. Men whose grip strength decreased over time had a 51 percent greater mortality risk compared with guys who maintained or increased strength. One possible reason: strength helps prevent disability and osteoporosis.

increased their midthigh muscle by 9 percent, and improved their walking speed by 48 percent. The message: It's never too late to adopt a healthy lifestyle.

## MYTH 3: EXERCISE ISN'T ENJOYABLE

***Reality Check:*** *It's important to find an activity that you like to do—you'll be much more likely to stick with it*

Jogging is one of the best ways to burn calories and condition your cardiovascular system, so it's worth trying to see if you like it. But it's not your only option. As we saw under Myth 1, the body burns calories with any kind of movement. Besides, if you have an aversion for an activity, how long are you going to keep at it, anyway?

The alternatives are many. You can bike outdoors or on a stationary bike; swim; walk; join a dance group; or play tennis or racquetball. Or do them all at different times in your life. Entrepreneur Susan Solovic mixes up her workouts, alternating between the treadmill and the elliptical trainer (where you stand upright and your feet move against resistance in an elliptical pattern). For even more variation, she goes walking outside or does yoga. "I believe in doing a variety of things so I don't get bored with any one routine," says Solovic, CEO and chairman of SBTV.com (Small Business Television), an internet-based television network for small businesses. "I think [boredom is] what causes people to fail."

## GOLF AS EXERCISE

Swedish researchers divided 19 male golfers by age—20s, 50s, and 70s—and monitored their heart rate while they walked an 18-hole round. The older the golfer, the more time he spent with a heart rate beating above 50 percent of his individual maximal heart rate. A day on the links corresponded to an exercise intensity that was moderate to high for older players, low to moderate for the middle-aged guys, and low for young golfers.

One of the points of exercise is to enjoy the sheer act of moving your arms, your legs, and your whole body—muscles, bones, joints, lungs, heart. You may remember that feeling from childhood—when it didn't matter if you were in a formal exercise program. Chances are, you just ran around and had fun. But as an adult—and especially living the life of an entrepreneur—it's easy to get lost in the cerebral side of your existence. By throwing yourself into the business, you may have lost touch with the simple joy in movement. And yet you remain a *physical* person who can find expression in *physical* action. Movement lets your body revel in that very real aspect of who you are.

## MYTH 4: A WOMAN WILL GET TOO BULKY IF SHE LIFTS WEIGHTS

***Reality Check:*** *Your body* will *change—you'll get more lean and flexible— but you won't get bulky*

This myth probably has its roots in the physiques of weight lifters such as strongmen, bodybuilders, and bruising National Football League linemen. So it's not really surprising that when you walk into any health club or gym, women are scarce in the dumbbell and barbell section. But the reality is that most women just don't have enough testosterone to pack on hefty muscles. This hormone is needed to increase protein synthesis, which leads to bigger muscles. Yes, it's true, because of genetic differences, that some women will be more apt to increase muscle size than others, but this won't be at all similar to the muscle increases men show. The

## WEIGHT TRAINING AND BONES

Lifting weights, or resistance training, doesn't just change your muscles—your bones also respond to the challenge by getting stronger and denser. In a 1995 study, researchers at the University of Arizona found increases of about 2 percent in bone-mineral density at the hip and lumbar spine after women age 28 to 39 did resistance training for 18 months. Older women have shown similar benefits from strength training. This is especially important given the prevalence of osteoporosis, a disease marked by low bone mass. Women make up 80 percent of the estimated 10 million Americans affected by the condition. (See Chapter 13 for more on osteoporosis.)

female bodybuilder physique is rare—these women have a genetic predisposition to build muscle and they do lots and lots of exercises. They also may take anabolic steroids and have abnormally low body fat percentages.

What a woman *can* expect from weight lifting is greater muscle strength—weight training makes her body better at recruiting muscle fibers to do an activity. A study from the 1970s found that weight-training women enjoyed strength gains ranging from 10 to 30 percent. At the same time, the women showed little overall increase in muscle size.

And while it's commonly thought that weight training makes you less flexible, the opposite actually is true. In another research study, ten weeks of strength training for women age 62 to 78 resulted in a 13 percent *increase* in their flexibility.

This increased strength and flexibility, of course, means everyday life is, well, just easier. Carrying a file down the hall, hauling groceries, picking up your kids, getting out of a car—all take strength. And the stronger you are, the less stress there is on your body.

## MYTH 5: EXERCISE IS DANGEROUS

***Reality Check:*** *Working out is safe when done with proper form, a moderate progression, and your doctor's clearance*

It's clear that physical *in*activity is a big risk to health. But what about the hazards of exercise—getting injured while lifting weights, getting into an accident, or suffering a medical emergency?

Of course, no activity is without its dangers. Even the proverbial crossing-of-the-street carries risks. But let's put this in perspective. While weight lifting certainly can lead to injury, this is largely avoidable—most injuries result from inexperience, improper form, or doing too much too soon. In reality, the rate of injury from training with weights and weight equipment is between 2.4 and 7.6 percent of participants in a given year.

That said, for someone with "silent atherosclerosis," or hardening of the arteries, vigorous exercise can bring on a heart attack in rare cases—so for anyone starting an exercise program, it's best to get your physician's clearance before going forward. Here's what the American Heart Association has to say on the subject: "The potential health benefits of exercise greatly outweigh the risk, although there is a very slight increased risk of death due to heart attack during vigorous exercise. Consult your doctor first if you have any concerns, have been sedentary, are overweight, are middle-aged or older, or have a medical condition."

## THE FACTS ABOUT FIXX

Some of the concerns about exercise and safety can no doubt be traced to Jim Fixx, the popular runner and writer who wrote a best-selling book on running in the 1970s. Fixx died tragically at the age of 52, suffering a heart attack while running. But what's probably not as well known is this: Fixx reportedly had a high heart disease risk because his father suffered a fatal heart attack at the age of 43. Fixx also was a former smoker with significantly high cholesterol, and had apparently ignored pain and discomfort in his chest. After his death, it was discovered that he had severe coronary artery disease.

## MYTH 6: IT TAKES TOO MUCH TIME TO EAT RIGHT AND EXERCISE

***Reality Check:*** *It doesn't take as much time as you may think*

One of the biggest misconceptions about physical activity is that it has to come all at once—the reality is that you can accumulate activity with short bouts throughout the day. In 2001, researchers reported in the *Journal of the American College of Nutrition* that either two bouts of 15 minutes or three bouts of 10 minutes result in similar aerobic benefits to 30 minutes of continuous activity. Also, another 2001 study, published in the journal *Health Psychology*, concluded that exercising for just 10 minutes improved mood, boosted vigor, and decreased fatigue.

And keep in mind that you don't have to make changes overnight—in fact, it's better if you make small incremental changes that will last. That means if you're sedentary now, you don't have to be jogging 30 minutes a day next week. Actually, you shouldn't be doing this. By approaching exercise in small chunks in the beginning, you can start stacking up successful workouts—building your confidence along the way and making it more likely that you'll stick with your new habit.

As for good nutrition, eating a healthy diet often just takes the split second required to make better food choices at the supermarket or a restaurant. For example, it takes no more time to pick up a few apples and oranges rather than grab a carton of cookie dough ice cream. It's no more trouble to throw a box of whole-grain cereal into your shopping cart instead of a box of Froot Loops.® The same goes for ordering the low-fat vinaigrette dressing at lunch rather than the full-fat

---

### TIME SAVER TIP

If you work at home and aren't seeing clients, put your workout clothes on when you get up in the morning, even if you're going to exercise in the afternoon. It will save time changing later and put you in a fitness mindset for the entire day.

blue cheese. Little choices like these throughout the week don't take any time but make big differences in the amount of calories you end up eating.

You don't even have to give up going to fast-food restaurants altogether. They shouldn't be a habit, but as with the grocery store and restaurants, it just takes making better choices—don't super size; instead of soda, drink nonfat milk; go for salads with light dressing and grilled chicken instead of the burger with cheese and bacon. (The Entrepreneur Diet in Chapter 7 has numerous smart fast-food choices.)

## TIME LINE

The latest government guidelines recommend a minimum of 30 minutes of moderate-intensity exercise most days of the week in order to reduce the risk of chronic diseases like coronary artery disease, type 2 diabetes, and colon cancer. To prevent weight gain, the guidelines suggest 60 minutes of moderate- to vigorous-intensity activity, and to sustain weight loss, 60 to 90 minutes of moderate-intensity activity.

While some have criticized these recommendations as excessive, keep in mind that activity is cumulative during the day. And remember that any activity is better than none. Here's a list of moderate and vigorous pursuits—but some activities can be either moderate or vigorous, depending on how hard or fast you go.

**Moderate**

- Hiking
- Light gardening/yard work
- Dancing
- Biking less than 10 mph
- Walking at 3.5 mph
- Light weight lifting
- Stretching

**Vigorous**

- Running at 5 mph
- Biking at more than 10 mph
- Swimming laps
- Aerobics
- Walking at 4.5 mph
- Heavy yard work, such as chopping wood
- Vigorous weight lifting
- Basketball

## MYTH 7: I WON'T BE ABLE TO ENJOY MY FAVORITE FOODS

***Reality Check:*** *As long as you have a generally healthy diet, occasional indulgences are OK, and there are ways to make your favorite dishes healthier and just as tasty*

If you believe this myth, you're not alone. In a national survey conducted by the American Dietetic Association in 1999, not wanting to forego favorite foods was the most frequent reason given by people who said they weren't doing anything more now than they were two years ago to eat a healthy diet. That's too bad, because this "all or nothing" attitude toward nutrition is self-defeating. You are not a machine, immune from the temptations of the chocolate mousse as the waiter wheels the dessert cart to your table.

But as long as you eat an overall healthy diet, there's nothing wrong with indulging occasionally. "There's no reason you have to give up hot fudge sundaes or french fries," registered dietitian Diane Quagliani said in a press release when announcing the American Dietetic Association survey results. "All foods can be a part of a healthful eating plan—it's all a matter of minding how often and how much you eat of some foods."

> *I believe in moderation—that you can eat meat, you can eat sweets, if you do it in moderation. It's just that the people who don't do it in moderation are the ones who get into trouble. My personal theory is to eat when you're hungry, not to eat out of habit.*
>
> —DOUG MACLEAN, CO-FOUNDER OF TALKING RAIN BEVERAGE COMPANY

### CAN EATING CAUSE YOU TO BURN CALORIES?

It's true: eating does burn calories. Actually, you burn calories even while you're resting—just maintaining the functioning of your body's systems requires energy. This "resting metabolism" represents between 65 to 70 percent of the total calories you expend in a day. Another 20 to 25 percent is spent in physical activity—although that number can increase if you're very active or decrease if you're sedentary. The rest—10 percent or so—is the result of the effort your body puts into eating and digesting your meals—called the "thermic effect of food."

It's also possible that eliminating all those enticing foods from your menu will make them all the more alluring, and you just may end up gorging if you can't stand it anymore. But by allowing yourself periodic "cheat" foods, you'll satisfy a craving in a controlled way.

Aside from treating yourself on occasion, there also are ways to make your favorite foods healthier—without sacrificing flavor. For tips on making small cooking tweaks that result in big health benefits, see executive chef Chad Luethje's advice in Appendix C.

## MYTH 8: NO PAIN, NO GAIN

***Reality Check:*** *While exercising may cause soreness, pain doesn't have to be part of your fitness routine*

With exercise, especially if you're new to it, there is some normal level of discomfort. After all, you're jolting your body from its resting state, making it jump into action, and causing changes all the way down to the cellular level. That's how your body gets stronger.

But just how intense and uncomfortable does exercise have to be? Activities that are intense or long in duration—such as running for a distance—can give health benefits beyond less-strenuous exercise. But the pace of a brisk walk is sufficient to boost the heart rate to a level benefiting overall health, according to researcher Kyle McInnis at the University of Massachusetts in Boston. When he asked obese men and women to maintain a "brisk but comfortable" pace while walking, the subjects all reached recommended exercise intensity levels.

"You really can get your heart rate up to the level that your doctor would recommend, and you don't have to jog or run to do it," McInnis said in 2003. "A large segment of the population still believes exercise must be vigorous, demanding, or involve more complicated activities than walking to adequately raise their heart rate. This perception of 'no pain, no gain' can discourage people from starting to exercise at all."

That's not to say that you won't feel some soreness after a workout (see the sidebar "Got DOMS?"). But be aware of pain caused by injury. "Good" soreness tends to be symmetrical—you'll feel it in both legs, say, from doing the squat exercise. "Bad" pain is typically on one side—your left knee, for example, after doing those squats.

## GOT DOMS?

Delayed onset muscle soreness, or DOMS, is common after a workout, especially if you haven't exercised before or are coming back after a long layoff. DOMS typically develops 12 hours or more after you exercise, and usually involves muscle soreness and stiffness that peaks in the first two days after your workout. The likely culprit is microscopic tearing of muscle fibers. But this breakdown is followed by rebuilding—and that's how your muscles grow and become stronger.

Ironically, exercise is a good way to alleviate DOMS pain. You can help minimize DOMS by always warming up and cooling down after your activity, and by not doing too much too soon. But it's important to go easy during your next workout and reduce intensity. You can also do exercises that target less DOMS-affected body parts to give your muscles time to recover.

Also, there's a difference between joint pain (not good) and muscle pain (usually OK). Joint pain tends to be very specific, and you'll know the exact spot that hurts—which usually is on or near the joint. Muscular pain is more diffuse.

## MYTH 9: IT'S INEVITABLE THAT I'LL GAIN WEIGHT AS I AGE, SO IT'S NOT WORTH FIGHTING IT

*Reality Check: Exercise can counteract the natural tendency to gain weight with age*

It's true we tend to put on pounds the older we get—at least in our middle years. Researchers at the University of Connecticut School of Medicine followed more than 5,000 Americans for 20 years starting in 1971, and found that people put on weight until middle age, stabilized, and then started to lose weight around the age of 60. The causes may include hormonal changes (for example, women undergo shifting levels of estrogen) and a genetic predisposition.

So if it can't be helped, why worry about it? Because other causes of age-related weight gain *are* under your control—one of the most important being strength

---

## BURNING OFF THE BELLY

Women in their late 60s who strength trained three times a week for 16 weeks showed nearly a 10 percent reduction in fat around the belly, which is linked with cardiovascular disease and type 2 diabetes.

---

training. From our mid-20s to our mid-50s, every year on average we lose one-half pound of muscle and add a pound of fat. Not good, when you consider that muscle tissue burns more calories than fat, and so our metabolism slows down by 5 percent every year.

But through resistance training, you can counteract that muscle atrophy and actually put on muscle. Add in other lifestyle changes—like aerobic exercise and eating wisely—and you'll defeat the middle-age spread.

### MYTH 10: I HAVE TO JOIN A GYM OR BUY EXPENSIVE EQUIPMENT TO GET IN SHAPE

***Reality Check:*** *You can exercise just about anywhere, anytime, and with minimal equipment*

Late-night infomercials want you to believe that fitness can be found in a contraption you can buy with three easy payments of $19.99. But exercise doesn't require complicated machines—you even can do some challenging exercises using just your body weight. Take Stephen Gatlin, founder and CEO of Gatlin Education Services. He's a regular runner, but he also adds push-ups to his fitness routine on a regular basis—"50 good, solid push-ups in a row," he says. "It doesn't do a whole lot of good to cheat yourself."

True, joining a gym can give you access to a personal trainer and plenty of weights and machines, and being around other people exercising can be a good source of motivation (more on this in Chapter 14). But working out at a health club isn't necessary to lead a healthy lifestyle. Stash a pair of dumbbells and a medicine ball under your office desk or in the garage, and you have a miniworkout facility at work or home.

Now that these health and fitness fictions have been uncovered, it's time to get started on the path to exercise and good nutrition. And the best place to begin is with a quick assessment of your current level of fitness.

---

### *Action* Items

➤ Take a minute to think about any preconceived ideas you may have about exercise or dieting. Did you learn them from reputable sources—for example, a physician, physical therapist, certified trainer, or registered dietitian? Or are they based on more shaky grounds, like a conversation you overheard at the gym?

➤ Take another minute to think about how these ideas may have played into your attitudes toward nutrition and working out. Have any of them kept you from starting on a healthy change in your lifestyle, such as lifting weights or eating a better overall diet?

---

# PART II

# *Start-Up*

# CHAPTER 4

# Taking Stock

*As a leader, as a CEO of a company that has 105 people working out of this office, I've got to be in good shape. I've got to look like I'm physically fit and on my game.*

—BRIAN SCUDAMORE, FOUNDER AND CEO OF 1-800-GOT-JUNK?

## ONE-MINUTE SUMMARY

🕐 By taking some basic health and fitness measurements, you'll know where you stand now and be able to mark your progress in the weeks ahead.

🕐 Important assessments include:

- Weight and body composition
- Cardiovascular conditioning
- Functional strength

🕐 Don't judge your results—simply observe and retest in four to six weeks to see how much progress you've made.

A balance sheet gives you a snapshot of how your business is doing at a particular point in time. Assets, liabilities, equity—all are laid out in plain view so you have a realistic appraisal of your success.

It's no different when it comes to your fitness. Just as you crunch the numbers to figure out the health of your business, now you'll take some measurements to find out the bottom line on the fitness of your body. And you can do it in about the time it takes to balance a checkbook. You evaluate several areas—weight and body composition, cardiovascular conditioning, and functional strength.

When you're beginning a new workout and nutrition program, assessing your fitness gives you a baseline measurement. As you progress in your program, you can periodically take these assessments again, charting your improvement and amping up your motivation—and if you persist, there *will* be improvement.

## THE INGREDIENTS OF FITNESS

Fitness is multidimensional, so it's important to look at it from different angles. That means considering things like how much fat your body carries, how strong your heart and lungs are, and how well your muscles function. Keep in mind that scoring low in one of these areas doesn't mean you can't score high in others. People tend to focus on one or two aspects—especially strength and aerobic ability—but this ignores the fact that other fitness elements also are important.

Take someone who runs a marathon—26.2 miles. She may be a great runner, but suppose her shoulder flexibility and strength are so low that she has trouble lifting a box overhead. You, on the other hand, may not be able to run a mile, but that box would be a piece of cake. So who's in better shape?

Since most of us have to lift boxes more often than we have to run 26 miles, you could argue that *you're* in better shape. But really, the point is to be aware that there isn't one dimension to fitness—and that you may already have strengths you aren't even aware of.

This chapter helps you figure out your strong points and weaknesses quickly—in about ten minutes, and with minimal equipment. Here's all you need:

- your height and weight,
- a tape measure,

- a calculator,
- a watch,
- a step about 12 inches high (or as near to this height as possible), and
- a full-length mirror

Use the Assessment Checklist on pages 61–62 at the end of the chapter to jot down your calculations. After you take the fitness snapshot of your physical assets and liabilities, you'll know the areas that you need to work on—and maybe some areas you can boast about.

## WEIGHT AND BODY COMPOSITION

To get an idea of how much weight, if any, you should lose, look at your current weight and "body composition." Body composition refers to how much of your body weight is fat vs. fat-free mass—which includes muscles, bones, tendons, and ligaments. And this calculation is important, because too much fat—particularly if it's centralized at your waist—puts you at greater health risk. First, we'll look at weight, then we'll consider body composition.

### *Weight*

For a general guide to determine your estimated target weight based on your frame size, use this formula.

- *Men.* Start with 106 pounds and add 6 pounds for every inch your height exceeds 5 feet.
- *Women.* Start with 100 pounds and add 5 pounds for every inch your height exceeds 5 feet.
- If you have a small frame, subtract 10 percent of the total pounds you calculated using the formula in the appropriate bullet above. If you have a large frame, add 10 percent. To estimate your frame size, circle your wrist with

> *I've been watching my diet more carefully of late, because now that I'm about to turn 58, I'd like to stay at 175 to 180 pounds, for my 5-foot-9½-inch frame. My body fat count is pretty good—it's probably about 12 or 13 percent.*
>
> —Stanley Wunderlich, chairman and CEO of Consulting for Strategic Growth 1 Ltd., an investor-relations company

your thumb and index finger. If the fingers overlap, you have a small frame; if they barely touch, you have a medium frame; and if they can't touch you have a large frame.

Record your current body weight and your estimated target weight in the Assessment Checklist at the end of the chapter.

### Body Composition

To find out whether you have a healthy body composition, use your body mass index (or BMI) and your waist circumference.

BODY MASS INDEX. BMI considers your weight in relation to your height, and for most people, BMI correlates closely with body fat. The more your BMI exceeds 25, the greater risk you may have of experiencing health issues. The number is calculated by dividing weight by height squared and multiplying by 703:

$$\frac{\text{Weight in pounds}\ \underline{\hspace{1cm}}}{(\text{Height in inches})^2\ \underline{\hspace{1cm}}} \quad \text{X} \quad 703 \quad = \quad \text{BMI}\ \underline{\hspace{1.5cm}}$$

A BMI of less than 18.5 is considered underweight, while a number from 25 to 29.9 is labeled overweight, and a BMI of 30 or more is categorized as obese. Keep in mind that this measurement isn't perfect—the BMI of someone with lots of muscle (such as an athlete) may be in the unhealthy category and yet his health risk generally is low. BMI measurements also have limitations with people who are less than 5 feet tall, senior citizens, and some racial and ethnic groups (such as African American and Hispanic/Latino American women).

You can also use Figure 4.1 to find your BMI category. Locate your weight at the bottom of the graph. Move straight up from there until you reach the line corresponding to your height. Record your results in the Assessment Checklist.

WAIST CIRCUMFERENCE. While BMI gives you a look at your overall body fat, *where* fat is located on your body can reveal health risks, even if your BMI is in the healthy range. Research indicates that people who carry fat mostly around their midsection (think "apple" shape) have a higher risk of cardiovascular disease,

FIGURE 4.1: **BMI Chart**

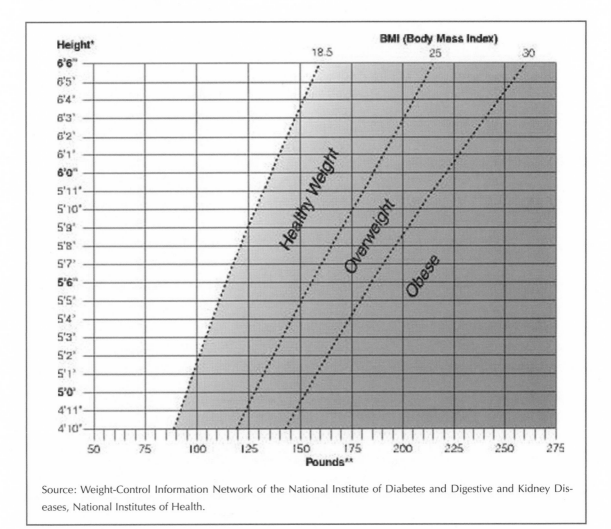

Source: Weight-Control Information Network of the National Institute of Diabetes and Digestive and Kidney Diseases, National Institutes of Health.

colon cancer, and diabetes than people whose fat is located in the hips and thighs (the "pear" shape). For women, a waist circumference greater than 35 inches, and for men a waist circumference greater than 40 inches, may increase disease risk. This is especially relevant for men, because they tend to carry their fat around the

## FIGURING FAT

Getting your body fat measured also can give you another way to evaluate your body composition. There are several methods used to get a reading, including:

- *Skin fold calipers.* A personal trainer or another health professional calculates body fat by pinching at various sites on the body to measure subcutaneous fat (the fat just beneath your skin).

- *Underwater weighing.* The concept is based on the idea that body fat floats, while muscle tends to sink. Check with the exercise physiology department of a local university to see if this test is available. FitnessWave offers mobile dunk tanks at health clubs in various states (http://getdunked.com).

- *Bioelectrical impedance.* This method uses an electrical signal passing through the body, based on the principles that muscle contains water and water conducts electricity. So the more muscle you have, the less resistance there will be to the current. Home devices include scales made by Tanita ($40 and up; www.tanita.com) and a hand-held version from Omron ($60; www.bodytrends.com).

Although there aren't any accepted standards for body fat percentage covering all ages, some researchers have recommended a range of 7 to 18 percent for active middle-aged men and 20 to 33 percent for active middle-aged women. Women with low body-fat percentages—18 percent or less—could develop amenorrhea, a serious condition causing menstruation to cease. Also, lower body fat in middle-aged women is linked to decreased bone density—a risk for osteoporosis. (See Chapter 13 for more on osteoporosis.)

belly. Women, on the other hand, are apt to have greater body fat than men but also are more likely to carry fat in the thighs and buttocks (although post-menopause some women tend to gain weight around the middle). So fat, it turns out, may be more risky for men than it is for women.

For this evaluation, simply use a tape measure to determine your waist circumference, measuring slightly above the hip bone (circling your bare abdomen) after you exhale. Make note of the result in the Assessment Checklist.

### *Look at All Your Measurements*

In order to assess where you stand, consider all three measurements (weight, BMI, and waist circumference), particularly your BMI and waist measurement. Having

---

## EXTRA CREDIT

Knowing some of your family's health history and getting some basic health readings can help you better clarify just how your weight may affect your health, according to the National Institutes of Health (NIH). With your doctor's help, determine if you have any of these risk factors:

- High blood pressure
- High LDL ("bad") cholesterol
- Low HDL ("good") cholesterol
- High triglycerides
- Elevated blood glucose (sugar)
- Family history of premature heart disease
- Physical inactivity
- Cigarette smoking

If you're considered overweight (a BMI of 25 to 29.9) or obese (a BMI of at least 30) and you have at least two of these risk factors, the NIH recommends weight loss. Losing just 10 percent of what you weigh now will reduce your disease risk.

But if you're in the overweight category, *and* your waist circumference is no more than 35 inches (women) or 40 inches (men), *and* you have fewer than two risk factors, you may be OK maintaining your current weight, according to NIH. Talk to your physician about your particular risk.

---

a large waist combined with a high BMI can make matters worse than having just one high measurement when it comes to the risks to your health.

Wherever your measurements fall, don't dwell on them. Like all these assessments, this isn't an opportunity to beat yourself up. It's simply a way to get a snapshot of where you are now. As you adopt healthier habits, when you check back in on your numbers, you'll be amazed at your improvement.

## CARDIOVASCULAR CONDITIONING

A muscle about the size of your fist, the heart beats a staggering 100,000 times a day. It coordinates with the lungs, veins, and arteries to keep your blood flowing throughout your body, day in and day out. And it does this all without any conscious effort on your part. Most of the time, you're not even aware of its work.

When you exercise—start a walking or jogging routine, let's say—your heart becomes better at what it does. In fact, one of the exciting things about beginning an exercise program is realizing the dynamic nature of your cardiovascular system—that it will adapt and improve itself in response to the work you give it. (More on this in Chapter 9).

Two measurements can give you a fast look at how well your cardio system is conditioned right now. Once you have these numbers, you can periodically recheck them to see how you're improving with exercise.

### Resting Heart Rate

Aerobic exercise increases your heart's ability to pump blood with each contraction. As a result, your resting heart rate typically slows down as your cardiovascular

## OVERTRAINING SIGNAL

In addition to using resting heart rate to gauge your fitness, you can use it as a tool to check if you're overdoing things once you start your fitness routine. If your resting heart rate is higher than normal, this can signal that you've overtrained your body and you need to take a day or two off from exercise.

---

**TIME SAVER TIP**

Even if you don't have time for a step test, still take your resting pulse—it's better than doing nothing, takes just a minute, and will give you some idea of where you stand.

---

fitness increases. In other words, the more fit you are, the less work your heart must perform to pump the same amount of blood.

The best time to take your resting heart rate is in the morning, just before getting out of bed (even when you're just sitting later in the day, your heart rate will tend to be higher than it is first thing in the morning). Measure your pulse at the wrist by firmly pressing your index and middle fingers on the inside of the opposite wrist, under the base of the thumb. Measure it for three mornings in a row, then record your average rate in the Assessment Checklist.

Normal resting heart rate is about 60 to 80 beats per minute (bpm), but in well-trained athletes it can be 40 to 60 bpm.

### *Three-Minute Step Test*

A step test is just what it sounds like—stepping up and down for three minutes. After you finish, measure your heart rate. Why is this a helpful test of fitness? Generally, a person with good cardiovascular power has a lower pulse rate immediately after exercise because his heart rate doesn't climb as much while doing the test and his pulse drops faster after he stops exercising.

HOW TO DO THE THREE-MINUTE STEP TEST. Find a sturdy step that's about 12 inches high (or the nearest equivalent), and start stepping—up with one foot followed by the other, then down with the lead foot followed by the other (that's one complete step). You should aim for 24 steps a minute, but just do the best you can and keep a regular pace by saying "up, up, down, down" or count out four beats.

When you finish after three minutes, immediately sit down and take your pulse for one minute—that's your score. Jot down your number in the Assessment Checklist and check how you've done based on the table in Figure 4.2.

FIGURE 4.2: **Three-Minute Step Test**

| MEN'S HEART RATE | | | | | | |
|---|---|---|---|---|---|---|
| **Age** | **18–25** | **26–35** | **36–45** | **46–55** | **56–65** | **>65** |
| **Excellent** | ≤76 | ≤76 | ≤76 | ≤82 | ≤77 | ≤81 |
| **Good** | 77–84 | 77–85 | 77–88 | 83–93 | 78–94 | 82–92 |
| **Above average** | 85–93 | 86–94 | 89–98 | 94–101 | 95–100 | 93–102 |
| **Average** | 94–100 | 95–102 | 99–105 | 102–111 | 101–109 | 103–110 |
| **Below average** | 101–107 | 103–110 | 106–113 | 112–119 | 110–117 | 111–118 |
| **Poor** | 108–119 | 111–121 | 114–124 | 120–126 | 118–128 | 119–126 |
| **Very poor** | ≥120 | ≥122 | ≥125 | ≥127 | ≥129 | ≥127 |

| WOMEN'S HEART RATE | | | | | | |
|---|---|---|---|---|---|---|
| **Age** | **18–25** | **26–35** | **36–45** | **46–55** | **56–65** | **>65** |
| **Excellent** | ≤81 | ≤80 | ≤84 | ≤91 | ≤92 | ≤92 |
| **Good** | 82–93 | 81–92 | 85–96 | 92–101 | 93–103 | 93–101 |
| **Above average** | 94–102 | 93–101 | 97–104 | 102–110 | 104–111 | 102–111 |
| **Average** | 103–110 | 102–110 | 105–112 | 111–118 | 112–118 | 112–121 |
| **Below average** | 111–120 | 111–119 | 113–120 | 119–124 | 119–127 | 122–126 |
| **Poor** | 121–131 | 120–129 | 121–132 | 125–132 | 128–135 | 127–133 |
| **Very poor** | ≥132 | ≥130 | ≥133 | ≥133 | ≥136 | ≥134 |

The test and data adapted from *YMCA Fitness Testing and Assessment Manual, 4th edition*, 2000, with permission of the YMCA of USA, Chicago, IL.

## FUNCTIONAL STRENGTH

Traditional bodybuilding programs have focused on building bigger muscles by doing exercises that tend to isolate particular parts of the body, and they don't typically challenge your ability to coordinate or balance. For example, a bench press is done by lying on a bench and pressing a barbell up and down.

But outside of a gym—in everyday life—the human body doesn't operate with isolated movements. The reality is that muscles, ligaments, bones, joints, and the nervous system interact so you can perform complex actions. Together these elements of your body form a "kinetic chain" that translates energy into movement.

Whenever you pick up a bag of groceries from your trunk or grab an extra-thick file out of the bottom drawer of your filing cabinet, you need good coordination, balance, and flexibility. So in becoming fit, developing bigger muscles is only part of the equation. You also need *functional* strength so that the elements of your body work together in the real world to make your movements fluid, more efficient, and less prone to injury.

There's an easy way to get a picture of your functional muscle strength, including your flexibility. The National Academy of Sports Medicine (NASM), an organization that certifies personal trainers, has developed an innovative fast-scan functional-movement assessment that looks at your posture as your body moves. Called the Overhead Squat Assessment, this lets you view certain "checkpoints" that signal how well all the elements of your body are working together.

---

### FUNCTION JUNCTION

A 2004 study at the University of Glasgow in Scotland put overweight women through a 12-week functional exercise program, working out twice a week for 40 minutes per session, and the results were impressive. Not only did the women show reductions in BMI and blood pressure, they also decreased the time it took to complete a 20-meter walk, lift a 1- and 2-kilogram bag onto a shelf, and climb stairs. The exercisers also boosted their score in a measurement of "life satisfaction."

---

"This assessment is the first thing that we look at from a musculoskeletal standpoint to address where a client's physical limitations are and what areas they need to work on," says Tyler Wallace, director of clinical services for NASM and a NASM performance-enhancement specialist and corrective-exercise specialist.

The idea is simple: As you squat, the various parts of your body (feet, knees, low back, shoulders, head) should maintain proper alignment. If they deviate—the knees buckle in or the back rounds, for example—then this is a sign that there is an imbalance, meaning muscle tightness or weakness around a joint.

How to Do the Overhead Squat Assessment. Preferably you should do this test barefoot. If you can, have a friend observe you and let her know what to look for. (See the Functional Strength section of the Assessment Checklist at the end of the chapter for cues to watch for.) All photos are courtesy of Karen Thomas of Entrepreneur Press and photographer Julia Cappelli.

1. Facing a full-length mirror, stand with your feet shoulder-width apart and toes pointed straight ahead.
2. Raise your arms straight above your head, fully extending your elbows. Your upper arms should be in line with your ears. (See Figure 4.3A.)
3. Keeping your arms above your head, squat down as if you were sitting in a chair, and then stand back up (see Figure 4.3B). Repeat the movement several times—observe yourself while facing the mirror, and then shift your body so you can get a view from the side (see Figure 4.3C).
4. Look for changes in the alignment of your feet, knees, low back, shoulders, and head (see Figures 4.4 and 4.5, for example). Record your observations in the Assessment Checklist at the end of the chapter.

Don't be concerned with how well you do—just note any deviations. The exercise plan in Chapter 8 and the flexibility program in Chapter 10 will take care of any imbalances.

FIGURE 4.3: **Overhead Squat Assessment**

A. Side View

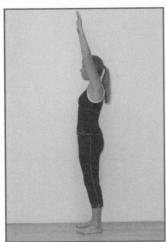

B. Front View

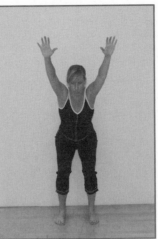

C. Side View

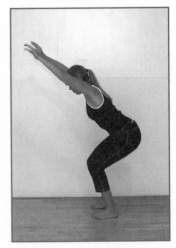

FIGURE 4.4: **Feet Flattened and Turned Out**

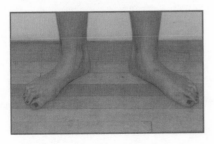

FIGURE 4.5: **Knees Buckled In**

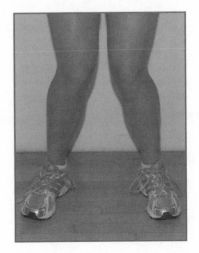

**FOR MORE INFORMATION ON ASSESSING YOUR HEALTH AND FITNESS**

In addition to the tests your physician takes, check your area for local health screenings and fairs, which can offer free blood pressure readings, body fat assessments, and other tests. You can also visit WebMD at www.webMD.com, which offers a BMI calculator and other assessment tools.

The purpose of the assessments in this chapter is to find out where you are now, so that in a short time you'll be able to see how far you've come. In general, it's a good idea to give your diet and exercise program a good four to six weeks before rechecking your assessment numbers (although it is OK to monitor your weight and waist circumference more regularly). Rest assured that with changes to your diet and activity levels, you'll make big strides.

---

### *Action* Items

➤ Complete the weight, body composition, cardiovascular conditioning, and functional strength tests, and fill in the Assessment Checklist. Retest in 6 weeks and 12 weeks.

➤ Just note how you do as a way to mark the progress you make; don't spend any energy judging your performance—save that for the exercises!

---

## ASSESSMENT CHECKLIST

**Your Measurements**

|  | **Baseline** | **+6 Weeks** | **+12 Weeks** |
|---|---|---|---|
| Weight | ____ | ____ | ____ |
| Estimated Target Weight | ____ | | |
| Body Composition | | | |
|   BMI | ____ | ____ | ____ |
|   Waist Circumference | ____ | ____ | ____ |
| Cardio Conditioning | | | |
|   Resting Heart Rate | ____ | ____ | ____ |
|   Three-Minute Step Test | ____ | ____ | ____ |

**Functional Strength**

*NASM Overhead Squat Assessment (recheck in four to six weeks)*

| Imbalance Checkpoints | What to look for | Yes | No | What it can mean |
|---|---|---|---|---|
| Feet | Feet turn out or arch flattens | | | Tight calf muscles, weak glutes (buttocks) |
| | Heels elevate | | | Tight calf muscles, weak shins |
| Knees | Knees buckle in | | | Tight inner thigh muscles and weak glutes |

| Imbalance Checkpoints | What to look for | Yes | No | What it can mean |
|---|---|---|---|---|
| Knees | Knees bow out | | | Tight hamstrings (the muscles in the back of your thighs) and weak glutes |
| Low back | Low back arches | | | Tight thigh or back muscles, weak glutes or low-back/hip/pelvic muscles |
| | Low back rounds | | | Tight hamstrings, weak glutes or low-back/hip/pelvic muscles |
| Shoulders | Arms fall forward or shoulders round | | | Tight chest and back muscles, weak back and shoulder muscles |
| Head | Head moves forward | | | Tight neck muscles |

# CHAPTER 5

# It's Time
# For a Change

*I hit my high weight and I said, "I'm going to change something."*

—Jon Lieb, founder and managing
director of Thirty Ink Media & Marketing

---

## ONE-MINUTE SUMMARY

- To make lasting change, you need to identify your underlying motivations for getting fit.
- You can best tap into these motivations by understanding the change process.
- Once you appreciate what's motivating you to get in shape, you can establish a vision statement for your health and fitness, and use the plans in the following chapters to get you there.
- Realize that lapses are a normal part of changing your behavior, but help minimize them by identifying "triggers" that knock you off course.
- Even when your new behavior is a habit, keep things fresh to avoid boredom.

Now that the assessment in Chapter 4 has given you an idea of where you are, it's a good time to figure out where you want to go. Taking just a few minutes to think about some of the things that are motivating you to lose weight or get fit can pay off in the long run. In fact, by understanding your motivators, you can tap into a powerful force that will keep driving you forward—which is especially important in the early going.

It's not enough to say, "I want to lose 20 pounds." This is why fad diets so often fail and the latest infomercial six-pack ab product collects dust in the den. At first blush, these diets and products are appealing because they seem to offer the "magic bullet" that will easily solve our weight issues. They may even work in the short run, and we may feel like we truly are changing.

But you must know why, really why, you want to make lifestyle changes. Without grasping the "why" of embarking on a health and fitness program, or anything else for that matter, you won't appreciate the underlying needs and emotions that are making you try in the first place. Plus, when you hit bumps in the road, it's too easy to give up. Your mind won't see the connection between the unpleasantness you're experiencing on the one hand and a meaningful reward on the other. You simply won't have the emotional attachment to your goals that can compel you to keep going through setbacks. You will be a sail without wind.

If you want lasting change, you must scratch the surface of why you're reading this book and take a closer look at what's underneath. You'll find a little self-reflection will go far. *This step, although it needn't take much time, is the most important aspect of getting fit and eating well.*

The best place to start is to understand how we go about changing a behavior in our lives. Then change becomes not a stressful event that happens *to* you but a process *you* control. And, most important, lasting, meaningful change becomes a reality.

## ALL THE WORLD IS IN A STAGE OF CHANGE

In recent years, experts in behavioral science have made important discoveries about how we change. Through their work with smoking cessation programs, James Prochaska, Ph.D., and Carlo DiClemente, Ph.D., developed a concept called the "Stages of Change" model. They determined that we progress through a series of identifiable steps on the road to a new behavior. The Stages of Change are precontemplation, contemplation, preparation, action, and maintenance. For any given behavior change, we are in one of these stages.

This theory has been found to apply in conquering alcohol addiction, undergoing dietary modifications, and adopting an exercise plan. In fact, Wellcoaches Corporation—an organization on the leading edge of the wellness movement that trains health professionals to coach clients in the areas of diet, fitness, stress, and overall health—has made the Stages of Change an important component of its work with clients (www.wellcoaches.com).

The basics of how people change seem to be similar across cultures in different parts of the world. And no doubt this predictable pattern of change applies to becoming an entrepreneur. As you read about the different stages below, think of how they may apply not just to healthy behavior but also to starting and running your business.

## PRECONTEMPLATION

In this stage, you're not yet thinking of changing your behavior. You're saying either "I won't" or "I can't." Because you've picked up this book, there's a good chance you've moved beyond this stage of change, but if not, keep in mind that precontemplation does not mean you can't change—it's simply a step on the road to new behavior.

Here are some tips for progressing beyond precontemplation.

- A person in this stage may lack enough knowledge to know how harmful a given behavior is, and so learning more about the detriments can help.
- Precontemplators may be rebelling—they don't want someone such as a well-meaning spouse or partner (or a pushy book!) telling them what to do. In this case, the person may find making smaller, incremental changes easier than abruptly changing—cutting down drinking at first rather than going abstinent, for example.
- A person may have a sense of hopelessness, resigned to failure because of past failures—someone, for example, who has tried multiple diets, meeting

with some success, only to gain the weight right back again. Understanding that relapses are perfectly normal can help this person view the experience as a learning opportunity, setting him up for success on his next attempt.

## CONTEMPLATION

In the contemplation stage, you start to give serious thought to changing a behavior, maybe gathering information about diets and exercise programs—such as taking a look at this book. But contemplation is not the same as commitment, and it's possible to spend months or years mired in this stage.

For example, workplace surveys indicate that up to 70 percent or more of smokers say they're interested in kicking the habit, yet when programs are put in place they typically attract 3 to 5 percent of smokers, according to William R. Miller, Ph.D. and Stephen Rollnick, Ph.D. Fully two-thirds of the population is in the contemplation stage when it comes to behavior change, says Margaret Moore, founder and CEO of Wellcoaches Corporation, herself an entrepreneur. "We have a world of chronic contemplators," she says.

> *To set goals, and to accomplish them, is a great thing.*
>
> —MARK ANDRUS, CO-FOUNDER OF STACY'S PITA CHIP COMPANY

The problem simply may be that you're ambivalent, and you've decided that the pros and cons of changing are pretty much equal. You realize that walking three days a week will help trim your waist and boost your energy, but on the other side of the ledger is the hassle of getting up a half hour earlier, or taking time away from your business commitments or your family.

If you've tried the Quick-Start Action Plan described in Chapter 2, that may be a good impetus to move you forward because you'll feel the benefits of a healthier lifestyle. Also, here are two helpful strategies to move beyond this stage and start taking action.

GO PRO. Focus on one or more pros that are particularly important to you—say, your long-term health or being a role model for your family or colleagues. Going over your fitness assessment from Chapter 4 or getting a checkup at the doctor can provide helpful feedback here (finding out your blood pressure and cholesterol levels, for example). This information is tangible and something you can relate to on a personal level, and can tip the pro/con balance in favor of positive change.

In a national study of people who successfully lost weight and kept it off for a year, the most common "trigger" event that led to the weight loss was medical related. And those who had medical reasons for losing weight dropped more pounds and had less weight regain over a two-year follow-up period. But don't wait until a medical emergency prompts you to action. See the health benefits ahead of time!

RATE YOUR READINESS. On the line below, mark where you are in your readiness to change your health and fitness.

not ready to change                                          ready to change

Now ask yourself, "Why didn't I place the mark farther to the left?" In other words, why do you have at least some inclination to change? In your answer, you'll discover some of your most potent motivators for change. Dig deep to find the underlying reasons. For example, motivators could include:

- I need more energy to handle the increasing demands of the business.
- I want to be more self-confident.
- I want to avoid the high blood pressure and heart disease that runs in my family.
- My spouse/partner is active, and I want to be able to keep pace.

Next, ask yourself, "What would it take to move the mark farther to the right?" Your answer will signal things you perceive as obstacles to change. Think about ways to overcome these hurdles, and be creative. If you feel you don't have time to go to the gym, for example, try bringing dumbbells to your office (you'll find a fast dumbbell workout in Chapter 8) or ask your employees to meet with you while you take a 15-minute walk. Consider asking an active client if he'd like to meet for a hike. If you find exercise boring, recruit your significant other or a friend to get involved and make it a social event.

---

### TIME SAVER TIP

Make exercise a family affair. "I use athletics as a social time," says Glenn Dietzel, a business consultant and CEO of AwakenTheAuthor Within.com. He incorporates family time by having his two sons ride their bikes while he and his wife go on a run. It's a win-win-win—his family's health benefits, he uses his time efficiently, and everyone has more fun.

---

In the blank lines at the end of the chapter, take a minute to jot down your motivators as well as your obstacles and the ways to get past them.

## PREPARATION

As you move past contemplation, you enter the preparation stage—you realize that you're ready to take action within the next month, although you still need to make a firm commitment. You may be in this stage right now when it comes to adopting a healthier lifestyle. Now is the time to express the vision of what you want to achieve and to make a plan to get there.

> *Part of the value of having a vision is that it helps articulate some of the innermost feelings of what the entrepreneur wants to achieve.*
>
> —Ray Smilor, Ph.D., executive director of the Beyster Institute at the Rady School, University of California San Diego and author of Daring Visionaries: How Entrepreneurs Build Companies, Inspire Allegiance, and Create Wealth

HAVING A VISION. Akin to a mission statement for your business, a vision statement for your health and fitness is a general assertion about where you'd like to be in six months or more *and, most important, why you want to be there.* This declaration gets to the heart of why you're trying to get fit, infusing your efforts with meaning and purpose. This goes behind the superficial "I want to lose weight" to articulate the root cause of your quest.

To do this, consider the motivations and obstacles you've listed. In thinking of your vision, areas

## WILLING, ABLE, AND READY

In the book *Motivational Interviewing: Preparing for Change, 2nd edition* (Guildford Press, 2002), William R. Miller, Ph.D. and Stephen Rollnick, Ph.D. say that you need to be willing, able, and ready to change.

### Willing

The change has to be important to you. The bigger the discrepancy between where you are now and where you'd like to be, the more important the change will seem and the more likely it is that your ambivalence will turn into resolve to change. So, for example, if you notice that your stamina is dragging during afternoon meetings, the image of yourself as a dynamic business leader isn't squaring with the reality of your energy slump—and so could provide an impetus to change.

### Able

You need to feel capable of the change. Smokers usually know all about the hazards of their habit and may consider quitting important, for example, but can feel that their chances of succeeding are just too low to even make the effort. Taking change in small, manageable steps can make earlier successes more likely and help give you a sense of confidence.

### Ready

You must place a high enough priority on the new behavior so that you want to start changing now. Losing weight may be important to you, and you may be confident you could do it, but it just may not be the most important change you want to tackle in the next several months. Listing your motivators in the worksheet at the end of the chapter will help make you ready.

you might cover include nutrition, exercise, and stress management. Focus on positive statements. As William R. Miller, Ph.D. and Stephen Rollnick, Ph.D. have written, "Constructive behavior change seems to arise when the person connects it with something of intrinsic value, something important, something cherished."

Or, as Wellcoaches' Margaret Moore puts it, "The foundation for lasting change is having our hearts working in sync with our heads and bodies."

Here are some examples of a health and fitness vision.

*My health and fitness vision . . .*

- in the next year is to lose the weight I've gained in the last several years so that I can feel younger and have a renewed sense of energy for my business.
- is to exercise regularly and bring my blood pressure and stress level under control in the next six months so that I'll be able to enjoy good health when I retire in five years.
- is to gain the stamina to hike the Inca Trail next year.
- is to adopt a regular exercise program and healthy eating habits so that I can inspire my employees and have more energy for my family.
- is to maintain a healthy weight and increase my endurance for long work-days.
- in the next eight months is to lose 20 pounds and build muscle so that I can improve my self-image and have more self-confidence.
- is to finish a 10K race six months from now so that I can have a challenging and competitive goal apart from my business achievements.

Just as your vision for your business is unique, so also is your vision for your health and fitness. And only you know what this is. Take a moment to write your vision statement in the worksheet at the end of the chapter.

PLANNING FOR SUCCESS. While your overall vision is the fuel that drives your change, an effective plan is the vehicle that will keep you rolling forward. Your vision statement is a broad view; planning gets down to specifics and keeps you focused. The following chapters help you do just that, giving you strategies for exercise, nutrition, stress management, and health.

> *Until one is committed, there is hesitancy, the chance to draw back . . . concerning all acts of initiative and creation. There is one elementary truth, the ignorance of which kills countless ideas and splendid plans: that the moment one definitely commits oneself, then Providence moves too. All sorts of things occur to help one that would never otherwise have occurred. A whole stream of events issues from the decision.*
>
> —JOHANN WOLFGANG VON GOETHE
> (1749–1832)

## MOUNTAIN MAN

For Jim Wilcher, the realization that he had to start paying more attention to his health came while he was still in his 20s. "I was going to school and building my business as a young man," he recalls, "and I wasn't very active." When Wilcher suffered chest pains and took a trip to the hospital, an intern told him he had suffered a heart attack.

"I remember lying on a gurney thinking that's it," he says now. "I've done all my skiing. I've done all those things I like to do, I'm done with it. That's it, for the rest of my life." Fortunately, as it turned out, Wilcher was suffering from a more benign, temporary condition known as pericarditis, which is inflammation around the heart.

But the experience, he says, was a wake-up call. He embarked on a fitness program, and today he is a dedicated runner and cyclist, sometimes biking as far as 200 miles a day. "I'm building a home gym now," says Wilcher, who lives near Seattle, Washington, and owns The Wilcher Group, an advertising, web development, and design business.

Wilcher has also summitted Mt. Rainier four times. Why mountain climbing? "I turned 40," Wilcher laughs, "and I decided I needed a different goal. I liked it so much, a group of friends and I kept doing it."

His activities, he says, provide a stress release to help handle the ups and downs of owning a business. He and an entrepreneur friend joke about "the monster" that can plague a business owner. "The monster," he says, "that comes and wakes you up about three in the morning and doesn't let you go back to sleep."

Wilcher calls on the memories of his mountain climbing and long bike rides to soothe his night-time worries. "As I'm lying in bed, I visualize myself actually getting out of my truck and loading my pack, or stepping onto my bike, and I retrace my entire journey as far as I can," he says. "And by the time I'm somewhere into the middle of it—I never get to the end—I'm asleep and back in the groove."

## ACTION

As you move from contemplation and begin to implement the strategies in this book, you are in the action stage of change, moving closer and closer to your vision.

It's important not to mistake action for permanent change. In this stage, there is a good chance of relapse—something that is completely normal. In fact, while it's possible to progress through the stages in order, relapses simply are part of the process of changing. Often, people who experience a relapse have better prospects of succeeding once they start again—they have minisuccesses that they can fall back on.

*I had stopped exercising because I was working about 100 hours a week. But I put the kibosh on that because I figured: one, I own the business, so there's no reason on earth that I should be doing this. And two, I had a client say to me: "Exercising is like brushing your teeth. You just have to do it. You have to make time for it." I started out by exercising just three days a week and allowing myself to sleep in on Tuesdays and Thursdays. Well, now I notice a huge difference in my energy. If I get up and exercise, I don't need caffeine during the day.*

—GINI DIETRICH, PRESIDENT OF THE PUBLIC RELATIONS FIRM ARMENT DIETRICH

That's why, as you go forward, it's a good idea to avoid an all-or-nothing mentality for your nutrition and exercise. If you miss two or three workouts, if you splurge on a large order of fries, don't get down on yourself. That can lead to a snowball effect where a relapse becomes a complete collapse. Know ahead of time—right now—that setbacks will happen and that's perfectly fine. *More so, setbacks are part of the process of change.*

At the same time, watch out for triggers that can set you back. For example, do you head to the vending machine for a Snickers® bar whenever you're about to have a meeting with a particularly troublesome client? Or do you grab a handful of M&M's® when it's time to get out the checkbook and pay vendor bills?

If so, these events are undercutting your efforts to get fit and eat well. They can happen at an almost subconscious level—you may think you're eating just because you're hungry, but the reality is that the snacks have become a way to deal with the stress of the moment. Your behavior is based on emotion—not physical hunger. Unfortunately, letting these

## OLD DOGS, NEW TRICKS

In understanding the Stages of Change, realize the importance of the power of your thoughts to change your health behavior. As mentioned in Chapter 1, contrary to the long-held belief that the brain's structure is rigid once we hit adulthood, neuroscientists are discovering that the brain remains much more flexible throughout life than was assumed.

In the book *The Mind and the Brain: Neuroplasticity and the Power of Mental Force* (HarperCollins, 2002), authors Jeffrey M. Schwartz, M.D., and Sharon Begley explain how the brain is able to rewire itself by making new neural connections. "We are seeing evidence of the brain's ability to remake itself throughout adult life, not only in response to outside stimuli but even in response to directed mental effort," they write. "We are seeing, in short, the brain's potential to correct its own flaws and enhance its own capacities."

In one experiment cited by Schwarz and Begley and originally reported in 1995 in the journal *Science*, the brains of people who started playing the violin even after the age of 12 assigned more neurons to the left hand's fingers. But the brain, it seems, also remodels itself based simply on our thoughts alone. So as you start to think increasingly like a person who eats well and exercises, your brain just may rewire itself to ensure that you really do.

triggers rule your day can leave you with a vague sense of lacking control—cascading down into a morass of more unhealthy behavior.

One way to identify your triggers is to jot down in a notebook when they occur and what kind of feelings or emotions you are experiencing. Keep a diary for five days, and then see if you notice any recurring patterns. By being more self-aware of trigger episodes, you can exert more control over your behavior.

## MAINTENANCE

This is the last stage in the change process and will hopefully last a lifetime. Now your new behavior has become habit, and you work to sustain the change. As routine sets in, you risk boredom, and so keeping your exercise and dietary changes fresh is important. In Chapter 14, you'll find ways to keep yourself on track.

With a good understanding of the change process and how to use the power of a vision statement, it's time to take action and begin to make your vision a reality.

---

### *Action* Items

➤ Think about what stage you are in when it comes to exercise, nutrition, and stress management (you could be in different stages for each), and what it might take to move you forward.

➤ Review what you wrote for your motivators, obstacles, and vision statement, and make sure your vision statement reflects your true reasons for wanting to change.

---

## MOTIVATION TO CHANGE WORKSHEET

When it comes to health and fitness, my motivators are:

_____

_____

_____

_____

The obstacles I may face, and the strategies to overcome them, are:

_____

_____

_____

_____

My health and fitness vision statement for the next ____ months is:

_____

_____

_____

_____

# PART III

# Building Your Body's Equity

# CHAPTER 6

# Eight Must-Have Nutrition Habits of Shedding Fat

*The key is to start with a healthy breakfast. I always have oatmeal handy—when I'm in a hurry in the morning, it's something I can heat up quickly.*

—MAX HOES, CO-OWNER OF CFR LINE, AN INTERNATIONAL TRANSPORTATION COMPANY SPECIALIZING IN OCEAN EXPORT OF AUTOMOBILES

---

**ONE-MINUTE SUMMARY**

- Fad diets fail because they don't offer lasting behavior change—the real secret behind successfully losing weight.
- There are eight key habits that promote weight loss. Each takes just a little thought to become a regular part of your daily diet.
    1. Don't skip meals
    2. Eat breakfast
    3. Control portion sizes
    4. Consume colorful fruits and veggies

5. Eat whole grains

6. Favor healthy fats

7. Cut down on added sugar

8. Aim for good, not perfect

The most popular diet at the turn of the 21st century was the Atkins Diet, a plan that called for eating few carbohydrates but plenty of high-protein, high-fat foods. Actually, the diet wasn't new—Robert Atkins, MD, had promoted the low-carb idea back in the 1970s. But as dieters became disillusioned with low-fat programs in the 1980s and 1990s, the Atkins approach regained a following, and then some. Low-carb offerings were popping up from fast-food meals to low-carb sodas and wines. Even fried chicken was being touted as a low-carb health food by one restaurant chain (until the Federal Trade Commission took notice).

But the low-carb fad turned out to be, well, a fad. In July 2005, Atkins Nutritionals, which marketed low-carb offerings, filed for Chapter 11 bankruptcy after losing $341 million the previous year. "Bankruptcy marks rapid fall of low-carb craze," read one August 2005 headline.

In the end, it may be that Atkins and its low-carb philosophy just couldn't deliver on the high expectations people had. True enough, low-carb diets can result in a quick weight loss initially. But much of this drop comes from water losses, and as the diet progresses, the average weekly weight loss is between one and two pounds—amounts seen in other diets.

Beyond Atkins, finding success with trendy diets can be elusive. Tufts-New England Medical Center did a one-year study analyzing the effectiveness of four popular diets—Atkins, Zone, Ornish, and Weight Watchers. The results were published in the *Journal of the American Medical Association* in 2005. At the end of the study, researchers reported, a quarter of the test subjects had dropped more than 5 percent of their weight—a small number even shed more than 10 percent.

But here's the other side of those stats—about 40 percent of the study participants quit the experiment before the year was up (the Atkins and Ornish plans saw the greatest percentage of dropouts). The most frequent reasons people gave for stopping were that a particular diet was too difficult to follow or that it wasn't producing results. Even many who stayed for the full length of the study adhered less and less to their diet over time.

Ultimately, it's easy to become bored with a diet and go back to your old eating habits, says Kathy Wise, a registered dietician and consultant who designed the exclusive Entrepreneur Diet and six-week meal plan for entrepreneurs you'll find in Chapter 7. "If there's no behavior modification," she says, "this can lead to yo-yo dieting, where you're on and off a diet. Each time you go through that cycle, you tend to get fatter than you were when you first started the diet."

If permanent weight loss and healthy eating are what you're after (you may have made this part of your vision statement in the previous chapter), then something more is needed—a shift in habits, not a quick fix diet. As entrepreneur Brian Scudamore, who lost 34 pounds by watching what he ate and exercising, puts it: "I don't feel like I'm on a crash diet. I feel like I've actually made a life change."

The eight behaviors given here are keys to making that lifestyle change, shedding excess pounds, and staying healthy. They take minimal time to implement, but like a solid business plan, these are the building blocks of good nutrition and weight management, rooted in the latest research. The Entrepreneur Diet in Chaper 7 is built on the foundation of these principles.

The more you take these ideas to heart, the more you'll discover that eating well becomes a natural, integral part of an overall healthy mindset, and that losing weight is an outcome not of denial but of affirming that you want the best for your mind and body.

## DON'T SKIP MEALS

Losing weight doesn't mean you have to starve yourself. In fact, going hungry is a sure way to *gain* weight. When you delay eating, your blood glucose (or sugar) levels drop too low, leading to a one-two punch of low energy and ravenous hunger. Your likely response: gorging on a large meal or running to the nearest vending machine to grab a candy bar for a quick, sugary fix.

You'll experience a fast energy boost—but at the cost of a sharp rise in blood glucose. This, in turn, causes the pancreas to release an extra helping of insulin, a

## MISSING MEALS

Swedish scientists found in a 2004 study that test subjects reported having significantly less energy and motivation at the close of the workday if they missed breakfast or lunch, or both.

hormone that helps shuttle all that glucose into your cells—including your fat cells. "If the body can't use all of the glucose for energy in the near term, it conserves it for later use by turning on the fat-storage mechanism," Wise says. "After years and years of doing this, we end up storing more fat than we ultimately need."

But the problems don't stop there. The insulin spike does such a good job of removing glucose from your blood stream that your blood sugar level falls below what it was before you ate. The result: your energy crashes, and you're hungry again, soon after your meal. That instant-energy candy bar has now caused the opposite of what you wanted—sluggishness.

*I think exercising, to some extent, helps you to be a better eater, because if you eat poorly for your dinner at night, you feel it the next morning when you get up to go running or hiking. So you're always thinking, "Well, I really want to hike tomorrow, and if I eat this I won't feel like doing that.*

—JENNIFER MELTON, CO-FOUNDER OF CLOUD STAR NATURAL PET PRODUCTS

But you can forgo these energy spikes and crashes by eating more frequent, balanced meals. That's why the Entrepreneur Diet calls for eating six times a day. By fueling your body about every three hours, you'll keep the blood-glucose levels more constant. "This will tend to control your cravings," Wise explains. "You're better able to regulate the amount of food that you eat and make better, healthier food choices."

## EAT BREAKFAST

This habit really could fall under the heading of "don't skip meals," but breakfast is so important, it deserves its own category. The National Weight Control Registry keeps track of thousands of people who have successfully lost weight and kept it off.

When looking at almost 3,000 people who each had lost at least 30 pounds and maintained it for at least a year, researchers found that 78 percent ate breakfast every day of the week, while about 90 percent ate breakfast on most days.

In addition to helping to stabilize blood sugar levels, eating a good breakfast sets you up for a healthy day. As a researcher at the Weight Control Registry, Holly Wyatt, M.D., said in the *Tufts University Health & Nutrition Letter,* October 2002: "When you start off your morning by eating a healthful breakfast, you are more likely to perform other good health behaviors, like taking a walk and eating lower fat foods."

## CONTROL PORTION SIZES

Managing portion sizes is a key to managing your weight. It's simple: If the food isn't in front of you, you can't eat it. And if it is on your plate, you more than likely will consume it. Research supports this idea. In a study published in 2005 in *Obesity Research*, one-half the subjects ate soup from regular bowls while the other half used modified bowls that were constantly refilled through a tube without the subjects' knowledge. The group eating from the bottomless bowls out-consumed those eating from regular bowls by eating 73 percent more soup and 113 more calories.

It's especially important to limit portion sizes on calorie-dense foods, such as cookies, rich spreads, cake, and other foods that trigger unhealthy eating patterns. Better yet, simply don't buy these temptations to have in your home or office, particularly in the early stages of losing weight.

Here are some more tips to keep in mind to help limit your portions:

- Use a salad plate for your main course, rather than a dinner plate. This switch can "trick" you into believing you're eating more food.
- If you're worried that you may not feel full with a smaller plate of food, include good amounts of vegetables and fruits, and start eating these first. They're low calorie and filling (more on this below), reducing the amount you eat of other, calorie-dense foods on your plate.
- Slow down. By eating slowly, you give your satiety mechanisms time to catch up to your food intake. In one small study reported in 2003, researchers at the University of Florida found that people who are obese may experience a delayed sense of fullness from eating—setting them up to overeat.

## GET THE FACTS STRAIGHT

Realize that the "serving size" given on a food's Nutrition Facts label is not an indication of how much you should eat. It's there to help you figure out the calories and nutrients in a given quantity of the food so you can compare it to similar products. When comparing two foods (say, two different types of cereal), first look at the serving size for each to see if you're comparing "apples to apples." Also, one package of food may contain multiple servings, so make sure to take this into account when figuring how many total calories and other nutrients are in the package.

- Avoid eating snacks out of the bag. Instead, take out a few chips or crackers and put them in a small bowl or on a napkin to help control your intake.

### CONSUME COLORFUL FRUITS AND VEGETABLES

Fruits and vegetables are full of water and fiber, making them high in volume but low in calories. Contrast this with other foods, say a slice of bacon or a cookie, which are low in volume but high in calories. Why is this important? Because *it's the volume of food, not the number of calories*, that gives us that full feeling and makes us stop eating, according to the Centers for Disease Control and Prevention. (Volume simply refers to how much space the food takes up in three dimensions.) So by substituting fruits and veggies for calorie-dense food (sorry, bacon and cookies count), you'll feel just as full but consume fewer calories.

Federal guidelines recommend five servings of veggies and four servings of fruit per day for a 2,000-calorie diet. A serving equals:

- ½ cup fresh, frozen, or canned fruit
- 1 medium fruit
- ¼ cup dried fruit
- ½ cup fruit juice
- ½ cup cut-up raw or cooked vegetables

---

**DARE TO COMPARE**

A one-ounce serving of corn chips contains about the same amount of calories as all these combined:

- one small apple
- one cup whole strawberries
- one cup carrots with 2 tablespoons low-fat dressing

---

- 1 cup raw leafy vegetables
- ½ cup vegetable juice

In choosing your fruits and veggies, aim for a variety of colors—reds, oranges, greens, yellows, blues, purples, whites (see "Power Foods"). Colorful veggies and fruit offer essential vitamins, minerals, fiber, and health-promoting substances called phytochemicals. There are hundreds of different phytochemicals, so don't focus on just one color group, advises 5-A-Day the Color Way, a partnership between governmental and industry groups. "By eating regularly from each color group," the organization reports, "you're giving yourself the widest health protection possible. Phytochemicals work together naturally in ways that supplements simply can't duplicate. For healthy results, whole foods are best."

Just make sure you're *substituting* fruits and veggies for less-healthy fare. If you simply add them on to your regular food intake, you could end up gaining weight.

## EAT WHOLE GRAINS

Research suggests that exchanging refined grains for whole grains may help battle overweight and obesity—one reason could be that the fiber helps you feel full. Whole grains also can help decrease coronary heart disease risk.

In fact, with research increasingly supporting the nutritional advantages of this food group, companies launched 183 new whole-grain offerings in the first part of 2005. Recent advances have allowed manufacturers to make tastier whole-grain

## POWER FOODS

Here's just a partial list of the powerhouse benefits of fruits and veggies. For more information, visit the Centers for Disease Control and Prevention web site at www.cdc.gov/nccdphp/dnpa/5aday and the 5-A-Day the Color Way web site at www.5aday.com.

- *Reds*. Contain lycopene, which may help combat heart disease and some cancers. Examples include tomatoes, watermelon, papaya, grapefruit, and guava.

- *Greens*. Carotenoids in spinach, kale, collards, and broccoli may promote eye health; cruciferous veggies such as cabbage, brussels sprouts, and kale are being researched to see if they decrease the risk of cancer.

- *Oranges*. Foods such as sweet potatoes, carrots, mangos, and apricots offer beta-carotene, a carotenoid that may boost immunity.

- *Yellows*. These contain lots of essential vitamins and carotenoids. Pineapples serve up manganese, vitamin C, and bromelain, a natural enzyme.

- *Blues/Purples*. Anthocyanins give off the blue color and may play a role in fending off carcinogens. Blueberries are high in vitamin C, folic acid, fiber, and potassium.

- *Whites*. Veggies such as onions, garlic, chives, scallions, and leeks contain allicin, a phytochemical that may benefit blood pressure and cholesterol. Cruciferous veggies such as cauliflower, as well as pears and green grapes, may help fight cancer.

pastas, and General Mills now uses whole grains in its "Big G" cereals—including Lucky Charms® and Golden Grahams®—although bear in mind that the sugar content may counter the healthy aspects of the whole grain, as pointed out in the July 2005 *Tufts University Health & Nutrition Letter*.

How do you know if a food is a whole-grain product? A grain qualifies as whole if, after processing, it still contains all three components of the plant seed—the bran, the germ, and the endosperm—in the original proportions found in the field, according to the Whole Grains Council, an industry organization.

Here are some facts about whole grains.

- The *bran* is the outer layer of the seed and contains antioxidants, fiber, and B vitamins.
- The *germ* is the part that can eventually grow into a new plant and offers B vitamins, minerals, protein, and healthy fats.
- The *endosperm* supplies energy to the germ, and contains carbohydrates, proteins, and small quantities of vitamins and minerals.
- Refining of grain leaves just the endosperm, with a loss of 17 nutrients and 25 percent of the grain's protein. Through processing, some vitamins and minerals are added back in, although fiber is not.

While most of us eat plenty of grains (such as bagels, cereals, rice, and pasta), we tend not to consume many whole-grain foods. At least half your grains should come from whole grains—and you need to be a smart shopper. Terms such as "multigrain," "stone-ground," "100% wheat," "cracked wheat," "seven grain," or "bran" typically do not refer to whole-grain foods, according to the U.S. Department of Agriculture. Make sure the first ingredient listed is a whole grain, as indicated by terms such as:

- Brown rice
- Bulgur
- Graham flour
- Whole-wheat flour
- Oatmeal
- Stone-ground whole (plus the name of the grain)
- Whole oats
- Whole rye
- Whole wheat
- Wild rice
- Whole-grain corn

## WHOLE-GRAIN SNACKS

For a quick and portable whole-grain snack, take along a small bag of whole-grain cereal, whole-wheat crackers, or baked tortilla chips. Another option: popcorn—it's a whole grain. Just nix the salt and butter.

## FAVOR HEALTHY FATS

Aside from making foods tastier, fat helps you feel satiated (and so less likely to overeat) and provides your body with energy—one gram of fat has nine calories, while a gram of carbohydrate or protein has just four calories. Fat also helps you absorb vitamins A, D, E, and K.

But not all fats are the same. Saturated and *trans* fat increase blood levels of LDL cholesterol, which is the "bad" cholesterol that raises the risk of heart disease. Trans fat offers a double whammy because it also lowers HDL cholesterol, the "good" cholesterol that prevents cholesterol build-up in the arteries. "While you should limit your intake of saturated fats," advises the Harvard School of Public Health, "it is important to eliminate trans fat from partially hydrogenated oils from your diet." The school cites one large study published in the journal *Lancet* in 1993 as finding that a daily substitution of just 30 calories of carbohydrates for 30 calories of trans fat almost doubled heart disease risk.

You'll find saturated fat in animal foods such as cheese, whole milk, butter, ice cream, and fatty meats. Trans fat, which is created when liquid vegetable oils are processed to become more solid, is contained in vegetable shortenings, some margarines, snack foods such as crackers and cookies, fried foods, doughnuts, baked goods, and other items containing partially hydrogenated oils. As of 2006, manufacturers must label the amount of trans fat in a food.

By contrast, unsaturated fats—known as monounsaturated or polyunsaturated fats—may lower LDL cholesterol and raise HDL cholesterol, although these "good" fats should still be eaten in moderation. Olive and canola oils are sources of monounsaturated fats, while polyunsaturated fats are found in nuts and fish, as well as corn, soybean, and sunflower oils (the "mono" and "poly" refer to the chemical composition of the fat).

The U.S. Food and Drug Administration's Center for Food Safety and Applied Nutrition web site (www.cfsan.fda.gov/~dms/transfat.html) has helpful tips in making smart choices about fat.

- When comparing similar foods, look at the food labels and add the saturated fat grams and the trans fat grams for each product. Also, check the percent Daily Value for cholesterol (as a rough guide, 5 percent Daily Value or less is low, 20 percent Daily Value or more is high). Choose the food that has the lowest numbers.

- Favor vegetable oils (but not palm kernal or coconut oils) and soft margarines (in liquid, tub, or spray form)—they're lower in trans fat, saturated fat, and cholesterol than are hard margarines and butter, according to the U.S. Food and Drug Administration. Virgin olive oil may be more heart-friendly than regular olive oil because it contains more polyphenols, an antioxidant, according to a study published in the *Annals of Internal Medicine*, September 2006.
- Try fish. Varieties such as sardines, mackerel, and salmon offer omega-3 fatty acids, which may fight heart disease.
- Choose lean meats and take the skin off poultry. For example, 3 ounces of pork loin is packed with protein while containing only 2.5 grams of saturated fat.

## CUT DOWN ON ADDED SUGAR

Reducing your intake of high-fructose corn syrup and other added sugars can quickly decrease your calorie consumption (and help avoid sharp rises and falls in insulin that may affect your energy levels). One of the best places to start is with sodas and fruit drinks. In the United States, the number-one source of added sugars is soft drinks. One 12-ounce soda boasts 150 calories and more than 40 grams of sugar. That's more than 10 teaspoons!

Sodas and sugar-added fruit drinks contain virtually no nutritional value, other than the sheer number of calories they put in your body. Add a daily soda on top of your current calorie intake and you'll gain 15 pounds in a year. In an eight-year study of more than 50,000 women, published in 2004 in the *Journal of the American Medical Association*, researchers found that drinking sugar-sweetened beverages was associated with increases in weight gain and risk of type 2 diabetes.

Many other processed foods contain good helpings of added sugars—some of the obvious include breakfast cereals, cookies, and yogurt. But other added sugar sources may surprise you—items such

> *I've cut sugar from my coffee, and I notice that I don't get a crash hitting me after the caffeine buzz dies down.*
>
> —DOMINIC RUBINO, OWNER OF FULCRUM AGENCY

## SOME KIND OF SYRUP

High-fructose corn syrup, or HFCS, is one of the most commonly added sugars, and manufacturers have increased its use in the last several decades as a less expensive way to sweeten food and beverages. HFCS accounted for about two calories per person per day in the U.S. food supply in 1970, while in 2004 it contributed almost 200 daily calories per person, according to a 2005 report from the U.S. Department of Agriculture Economic Research Service. In fact, the rise in HFCS has corresponded with the increase in obesity in the United States, and one theory is that the body metabolizes fructose differently than other added sugars, promoting extra body fat and a boost in appetite. (Still, the evidence is insufficient at this point to blame HFCS, according to the American Dietetic Association.)

as ketchup, soup, barbeque sauce, salad dressing, peanut butter, and granola bars. No wonder that by the year 2000, Americans on average were eating more than twice the recommended amount of added sugars, according to the American Dietetic Association. "The problem is," the association reports, "sugar can add 'empty' calories and displace other, more nutritious foods."

Read the Nutrition Facts label on foods, which lists "total sugar" in grams. This includes natural and added sugar, but if sugar is high on the list of ingredients, it's likely that most of it is added. Names to look for include:

- Sugar (brown, white, raw, or cane)
- Corn sweetener, corn syrup, high-fructose corn syrup
- Dextrose, fructose, sucrose, glucose, lactose, maltose
- Molasses, honey
- Fruit juice concentrate

It's best to limit added sugars to less than 10 percent of your total daily calories, but this isn't easy. Consume one 12-ounce soda (about 150 calories and around 10 teaspoons of sugar) and you're almost at your limit. But there are ways to cut down.

- Eliminate sugary drinks, or at least begin to reduce your consumption. If you drink two sodas per day, reduce it to one. Ditto for fruit punch or fruit "cocktail" drinks. Better yet replace these beverages with water or a mixture of club soda with orange juice or a squeeze of lime.

- Switch your regular sugary cereal for one with 8 grams of sugar or fewer per serving.
- Don't be fooled by fat-free foods. No-fat cookies, ice cream, and other foods may contain the same amount of sugar as the full-fat varieties and can be calorie rich.
- Substitute fruit for candy, high-fat granola bars, cakes, and other baked sweets.

## AIM FOR GOOD, NOT PERFECT

You may think that right now just isn't the best time to get your nutrition on track. Your business has you working long hours plus you've got family and personal commitments. You just won't be able to give 100 percent to a diet at this point—so it's better to put it off.

### SUGAR SUBSTITUTES

Food manufacturers recently have flooded stores with new products touting no and low sugar, sweetened by sugar substitutes, such as sucralose (called Splenda®). "Low-sugar has become the new low-carb," reported a 2005 story in *The New York Times*. Many experts say artificial sweeteners are a good way to reduce sugar and calories, but "some critics voice concern about the increased consumption of what are essentially chemical sweeteners, especially among children," *The Times* reported. The article also cited the marketer of Splenda referring to numerous studies confirming safety. Another *Times* article, in 2006, reported on research indicating that aspartame (sold as NutraSweet® and Equal®) was associated with cancers in rats. But in April 2006, the *Associated Press* reported that a newly announced study by National Cancer Institute scientists on hundreds of thousands of people age 50 to 69 found no increased cancer risk from aspartame consumption. Whatever the merits of the debate on the health aspects of artificial sweeteners, realize that some reduced-sugar items actually offer the same number of calories as in their original form. And artificial sweeteners won't do anything to curb your sugar cravings. If you use them, do so sparingly and try fruit instead to satisfy your sweet tooth.

Take the advice of the philosopher Voltaire—to paraphrase, don't let "perfect" be the enemy of "good." In other words, you may not be able to give a diet your absolute best shot right now, but you can do *something*. That something will be an improvement. Maybe not perfect, but better.

Also remember that there will be times when you stray from your diet, when you give in to the temptations of, say, a half a box of chocolates. You have a choice when this happens, explains nutritionist Kathy Wise—you can throw up your hands and say: "I've messed up, so I may as well forget this diet thing. Gimme the rest of that box." Or, you can give yourself a break and take something positive away from the experience.

For example, if it was a stressful business phone call that set off your eating, ask yourself if the chocolate helped the situation. "Don't beat yourself up when you make a mistake," Wise advises. "Learn from it and ask yourself, 'All right, what happened, how did it happen, and what would I do differently next time?'"

And remember, figure you're not perfect but you're still good, and move on.

---

### *Action* Items

➤ Take a minute to think about what kind of good or bad habits you may have when it comes to food. For example, do you always make a point to eat a healthy breakfast? Do you get so wrapped up in work that you forget to eat, and then just grab a candy bar and a soft drink?

➤ Take another minute to think about times when you may have been stressed and you turned to food. Did it make you feel calmer? Was there some other way you could have managed the stress? (Look for stress management techniques in Chapter 11.)

---

# CHAPTER 7

# The Entrepreneur Diet

*When you're 46 years old and you let your diet go too much, it goes to your waist in a heartbeat. And it's hard to get rid of. So I've just been careful about it and set the weight that I like and feel comfortable at, and that's the weight I stay at.*

—Dan Santy, founder of Santy Advertising

## ONE-MINUTE SUMMARY

- The Entrepreneur Diet is exclusively designed with the time-crunched entrepreneur in mind, while also incorporating the eight must-have nutrition habits described in Chapter 6.
- The diet is easy to use and will keep you energized throughout the day, delivering lasting weight-loss results.
- The diet is flexible—you can repeat the same day's menu several days in a row, or mix and match your favorite meals.

With long hours devoted to building your company, you don't have time for complicated meal plans or counting calories. Instead, you need a practical nutrition guide that focuses on the unique challenges you face as a business owner, while also offering lasting weight loss.

With that in mind, registered dietician and wellness coach Kathy Wise has exclusively designed an innovative, no-hassle six-week menu plan for an entrepreneur on the go. Based on the eight must-have nutrition habits described in Chapter 6 as well as her years of experience helping businesspeople reach their weight loss goals, Wise's program is

- *time efficient*—featuring quick, easy-to-prepare meals and snacks.
- *energy enhancing*—minimizing hunger pangs while promoting stable blood-sugar levels throughout the day so you can maintain sharp focus and energy for the demands of your business.
- *flexible and practical*—including fast-food, frozen entrée, and restaurant alternatives so you can make healthy food choices and stay on track no matter where you are.
- *sensible*—featuring a balance of carbohydrates, protein, and healthy fats, as well as whole grains, fruits, veggies, and lean meats.
- *results-driven*—targeting consistent and healthy weight loss of between one and two pounds a week.

"As an entrepreneur myself, I know how difficult it is to maintain a healthy diet when your business demands so much of your time and attention," Wise says. "So I tailor made this meal plan for the entrepreneur by making it as flexible and easy-to-use as possible."

This chapter outlines how to make the Entrepreneur Diet work for you.

## ADJUST THE PLAN TO YOUR WEIGHT

The diet calls for eating about 1,700 to 1,750 calories per day, which will promote fat loss for a person who weighs 180 pounds or more. If you weigh less, simply reduce portion sizes across the board—or if you want to be more precise, you can easily adjust the amount of food you should eat based on your own weight. Here's how:

## NUTRITIONIST AS ENTREPRENEUR

Registered dietitian Kathy Wise, who designed the Entrepreneur Diet, decided early in life to gain control over her weight. "I was an obese child with an overweight mother and grandmother," she says. "I hated being overweight and disliked the way I felt about myself. I watched my grandmother have her weight interfere with her life and health and my mom bounce from diet to diet." She decided to change her future and avoid becoming an obese adult. "I started to watch my diet and exercise," she remembers. "I lost about 50 pounds and felt so great about myself and my life that I decided I would never be overweight or out of shape again."

In her college years, she worked as an aerobic and exercise instructor, and ended up fielding lots of nutrition questions from her students—prompting her to change her major to nutrition and dietetics.

After working as a hospital dietitian, she launched her own full-time consulting business in 1997 (she now serves on the executive board of the American Dietetic Association's Entrepreneurs Practice Group). "I enjoy being in charge of my life and my income, and being able to decide where I want to concentrate my efforts," she says. "I love having my clients satisfied and helping them attain their health and wellness goals."

Wise's own workout routine includes daily runs of between three and five miles and strength training three times per week. In addition, good nutrition, she says, benefits her business pursuits. "I use my diet to keep energized and thinking sharp," she says. "My own nutrition helps me work long hours and still have energy to work out and have fun with family and friends. I am a 'product of my product,' which sets a good example for my clients and helps establish credibility."

If you're launching a consulting business, start with a business plan—even if you're not going to borrow start-up money, advises Wise. "Your plan will be your road map to guide you in making business decisions," she says. "It will help you decide who your clients will be and how you'll attain and maintain them, as well as keep you focused on your goals."

You can contact Wise through her web site at www.nutrawise.com.

- *If you are between 150 and 180 pounds.* Omit the dinner carbohydrate (i.e., the potato, rice, pasta, or bread). For example, skip the sweet potato for the dinner meal on Day 1, the brown rice for the dinner meal on Day 2, and so on.
- *If you are below 150 pounds.* Omit the dinner carbohydrate *plus* cut the dinner protein (i.e., meat or fish) in half (to 3 or 4 ounces) *plus* omit the mid-morning snack. When eating at a restaurant, cut the portion size of the entire meal in half.

## KNOW PORTION SIZES

You can eyeball portion sizes—there's no need to measure out cups, ounces, and tablespoons. Below is a quick-reference guide that gives you common objects to use as a guideline when figuring the amount of food you're eating. (If you've got the time and inclination, then by all means take out the cups and spoons, and measure ingredients for the first few days to get an even better feel for the portions sizes.)

### Common Measurements

1 cup vegetables, fruit, pasta, cottage cheese, oatmeal = average adult fist

½ cup applesauce, yogurt = tennis ball

3 ounces meat = deck of cards, palm of hand, or bar of soap

3 ounces fish = checkbook

1 ounce nuts or trail mix = surface of 1 adult palm

1 ounce cheese = 4 dice, a thumb or 2 dominoes

1 tablespoon peanut butter = ½ ping-pong ball

1 teaspoon reduced-fat mayo or low-fat salad dressing = tip of thumb

1 bagel = slightly larger than a compact disc

Comparison information was compiled from the American Cancer Society; Susan E. Gebhardt and Robin G. Thomas's "Nutritive Value of Foods" (U.S. Department of Agriculture); and the National Dairy Council.

## EXPECT TO LOSE ONE TO TWO POUNDS A WEEK

Generally, this is a safe and realistic rate of weight loss when you're reducing your calories and exercising. Your actual rate of weight loss will depend on your metabolism

## IN PRAISE OF THE TV DINNER

Frozen meals have a built-in fat loss advantage—portion control. In fact, in a study published in 2004 in *Obesity Research*, researchers found that women who ate two daily frozen entrées from Uncle Ben's (which sponsored the study) lost more weight and body fat than women who ate a similar diet but without the frozen meals.

(how efficient your body is at burning the calories you take in). Daily fluctuations in weight are common so weigh yourself no more than once a week. You can also track your progress by simply checking how your clothes are fitting and by measuring your waist with a tape measure—again no more than one time per week (you'll also do this as part of your periodic health and fitness measurements described in Chapter 4).

Once you hit your goal weight, you can add a second afternoon snack—just keep monitoring your weight and waist circumference on a weekly basis until you have a good feel that you're sustaining your weight loss.

## TIME YOUR WORKOUTS

Scheduling a workout within a short time after one of the menu's snacks will provide a good source of energy, without taking away too much of your body's resources for digestion. For this reason, try to avoid scheduling your walks, runs, or resistance exercise sessions shortly after eating one of the three bigger meals of the day.

## STAY FLEXIBLE

The plan is not meant to be a rigid blueprint that you have to follow to the letter. You can certainly do so, but if you prefer, you can simply choose one of the days you particularly like and repeat it for several days before moving to another day. You can also modify the plan by mixing meals from various days—say, breakfast

---

**A WORD OF CAUTION**

Before modifying your diet, check with your doctor, particularly if you have a history of any health concerns. Also, there are multiple fish servings in the meal plan; the government has advised pregnant women, those who may become pregnant, nursing mothers, and young children to avoid some types of fish (including swordfish) and to limit other fish and shellfish to 12 ounces a week (albacore tuna should be limited to 6 ounces per week because it contains more mercury than canned light tuna). For more information, visit www.cfsan.fda.gov/~dms/admehg3.html.

and midmorning snack from Day 1, lunch and midafternoon snack from Day 2, dinner and evening snack from Day 4. And if you're short on time, there are "Quick Fix" alternatives for breakfast, lunch, dinner, and snacks, as well as restaurant options. With all of the choices the menu offers, you're bound to find plenty of meals that appeal to your palette.

## HYDRATE

Stay well-hydrated during the day. Sipping on ice water (or a warm cup of tea, if you prefer) may give you a sense of fullness if you have hunger pangs and help you avoid mindlessly munching on food when you're in the middle of an all-consuming business project.

**TIME SAVER TIP**

The meal plan often includes an option of using a "ready to drink" shake of protein and carbohydrate for one of your daily snacks. These are quick and ideal low-fat meals on the go.

## PLAN AHEAD

Try to prepare your meals the night before—in the morning rush, it's too easy to run out of time. Take a weekly trip to the grocery store to make sure you've got all the supplies required for the next week. Getting the bulk of your shopping done in one trip with a clear purpose will save time and reduce the chances you'll succumb to a junk food meal midweek. Lastly, purchase a good-sized insulated lunch bag for packing your meals—both when you head to work and for travel.

## START SMALL

If you're not ready to commit to the six-week meal plan of the Entrepreneur Diet, it's fine to begin with small steps if that's what you're ready for. Look at your worst habit and start there, Wise advises. "If you never eat breakfast, for example, simply try to eat a healthy morning meal every day this next week," she explains. By making these more manageable changes, success will breed success. And as you gain confidence, you can try for more—including the six-week meal plan.

## BE A SMART SHOPPER

- Don't go to the grocery store on an empty stomach, and make a shopping list—you'll be less likely to impulse buy unhealthy foods.

- Favor natural foods while reducing your purchases of processed foods.

- Look at the Nutrition Facts label when comparing foods. Check the percent Daily Value when available—5 percent Daily Value or less is low, while 20 percent Daily Value or more is high, according to the USDA's web site www.nutrition.gov. Look for a low percent Daily Value of saturated fats, trans fat, cholesterol, and sodium. The percent Daily Value should be higher for fiber; vitamins A, C, and E; potassium; magnesium; calcium; and iron.

- Visit a farmers' market, where you can buy fresh produce and other good-for-you foods. To locate a market in your area, visit www.ams.usda.gov/farmersmarkets/map.htm.

## THE CALORIC COST OF ALCOHOL

When you go out for drinks with a client, sip wine with dinner, or just relax with a beer when you get home, you're adding extra calories to your day. Just how many depends on the type of alcohol you're drinking. While alcohol in moderation may confer some health benefits (see Chapter 13), keep in mind that a regular habit can add up over time. Averaging four regular beers a week will mean almost 2,400 extra calories a month or more than 28,000 a year. That translates to eight added pounds on your scale. Do that for five years and, well, you get the picture. What's more, research indicates that alcohol may stimulate appetite, possibly by inhibiting secretion of leptin, a hormone that is important in appetite regulation.

Remember that juices, sodas, and syrups added to drinks boost calorie content. If you do imbibe, this chart shows you which drinks carry the most calories so you can make smart choices (numbers are approximate and vary by brand).

| Beverage | Serving Amount | Calories |
|---|---|---|
| Margarita | 5 ounces | 550 |
| Martini | 5 ounces | 343 |
| Piña colada | 5 ounces | 273 |
| Long Island ice tea | 5 ounces | 238 |
| Beer (regular) | 12 ounces | 149 |
| Red wine (Zinfandel) | 5 ounces | 131 |
| Red wine (Burgundy) | 5 ounces | 129 |
| White wine (Pinot Grigio) | 5 ounces | 123 |
| Gin | 1½-ounce jigger | 116 |
| Rum | 1½-ounce jigger | 116 |
| Vodka | 1½-ounce jigger | 116 |
| Whiskey | 1½-ounce jigger | 116 |
| Beer (light) | 12 ounces | 110 |

Information compiled from the National Instititue on Alchohol Abuse and Alcoholism at www.collegdrinkingpreven tion.gov; the McKinley Health Center, University of Illinois at Urbana-Champaign at www.mckinley.uiuc.edu/hand outs/alcohol_nutrit_101.html; and the USDA Nutrient Data Laboratory at www.nal.usda.gov/fnic/foodcomp/search/.

## GIVE YOURSELF A BREAK

Don't have an all-or-nothing approach to the meal plan—in fact, it's fine to splurge occasionally on your favorite food. A rigid attitude is counterproductive in the long run—by constantly denying yourself, it's a lot less likely you'll stick with the plan. A diet isn't about deprivation; it's about making wiser choices over time so that your overall eating pattern becomes healthier. It's unrealistic to think that every nutrition step you take will be in the right direction. Good nutrition doesn't have to move in a straight line—but over time, your food choices will become better and better.

---

### *Action* Items

➤ Read through the six-week meal plan to get a feel for the types and amounts of foods you'll eat.

➤ Plan a trip to the grocery store in the next week to pick up the meal-plan items you'll need in the first week or so.

➤ Take a minute to think about recent business lunches or dinners you've had. Did you overeat or order unhealthy items?

---

## THE ENTREPRENEUR DIET SIX-WEEK MEAL PLAN

The following pages contain a six-week diet designed exclusively by nutrition expert Kathy Wise, R.D. The meal plan will help you implement the nutrition principles in this book in a practical, no-hassle way. Rather than focusing on precise breakdowns of how much of each meal comes from fat, protein, and carbohydrates, the menu is based on an overall healthy balance among these nutrients. Also, the plan is based on an average calorie intake—some days you'll take in a little more; on others you'll eat a little less.

Here are quick highlights to keep in mind:

- The meal plan includes many frozen dinners and fast foods to keep you eating well on-the-go. These are not ideal meals to eat on a regular basis—they can be very high in sodium, for example. But when you're time-crunched, you have to make choices among less-than-perfect alternatives. These options are meant to give you the best selections when you're eating out or don't have time to prepare a more involved meal at home. And always check to see if a restaurant has a "fit"-type of menu. Just remember that moderation is important—as much as possible, focus on eating home-prepared foods instead.

- For the power shakes listed, use about 25 grams of protein per shake (usually this will be a little more than one scoop of protein powder, but check the label). Look for protein powder products that contain whey protein isolate, which offers high levels of branched chain amino acids—these are important in helping build muscle.

- Light margarine is used in many of the meals. Choose products that list zero trans fat on the nutrition label. (Although even with these products you may see the words "partially hydrogenated" in the list of ingredients. This is because if the level of trans fat is less than .5 grams the manufacturer can say the product is trans-fat free). If you prefer to use olive oil in place of light margarine, then limit it to half the amount of light margarine to keep the calories about the same (for example, 1 T. olive oil instead of 2 T. light margarine). A calorie-free option is nonstick cooking spray.

- To lower your cholesterol intake, use an egg substitute in preparing the scrambled egg and omelet meals.

- "T." stands for tablespoon, while "t." signifies teaspoon. "Light" yogurt refers to low-sugar varieties such as Dannon® Lite 'n Fit™. For "lean" meats, look for foods that contain 10 percent or less fat, or that show minimal marbling fat (fat woven within the meat). You should also trim visible fat. For "sautéed" foods, use a skillet and cook over high heat for just a few minutes.

- Red Bull Energy Drink is listed in the snack category—this, or a similar energy drink, can be an effective way to boost your energy shortly before a workout. Just remember that these beverages contain caffeine and may not

## VICTORY OVER THE VENDING MACHINE

Vending machines tend to carry junk food, so it's best to steer clear. But they're so convenient that it's likely you'll be pushing a button or two in the days ahead. The good news is that vending distributors are starting to offer healthier choices. Still, be on your toes. Look for baked chips, dried or regular fruit, light yogurt, pretzels, or nuts (roasted or raw varieties, and not salted or honey-roasted nuts). Nonfat milk is a good source of calcium and protein. Avoid cakes, cookies, regular chips, donuts, and candy bars, which provide high calories, fat (including trans fat in some cases), and sugar. Choose diet soda over regular soda, take the cheese off of sandwiches, and shun chicken, tuna, or egg salad sandwiches (they could very likely be made with full-fat mayonnaise). Don't be fooled by fruit juices—watch out for added sugar and look for 100 percent real juice. And if you just must have chocolate, opt for dark chocolate, which offers flavanols, compounds that help produce nitric oxide in the blood and decrease blood pressure.

be appropriate for some people (including pregnant or nursing mothers and those with heart conditions).

- Some products listed may not be in some grocery stores—try markets that carry natural and organic foods such as Trader Joe's and Whole Foods Markets®.
- Some meals include drinks, but many do not. To keep calorie counts the same as listed—and boost health—remember that ice water is an excellent, healthy choice, as is tea or sparkling water. Diet colas are another, less desirable alternative. Keep in mind that adding a glass of wine to a meal will add about 130 calories to your day's total, while a 12-ounce soft drink will tack on 150 calories. If you do include these types of beverages, try to do so on days when you're eating lower-calorie meals.
- Recall, as mentioned earlier in the chapter, that days and meals of the plan are meant to be flexible and interchangeable. You can repeat one of your favorite days several times, and you can interchange meals from different days (i.e., lunch from Week Two, Day Three with lunch from Week Two, Day Five).

Enjoy!

# WEEK ONE, DAY ONE

**Breakfast** _____ or _____ **Quick Fix Breakfast**

Power shake: Mix 1 scoop whey protein
powder, 1 c. pineapple, ½ c. low-fat
vanilla yogurt, and 1 c. nonfat milk

Calories: 325, Protein: 35g, Carbohydrate: 43g, Fat: 1g

Starbucks® Biscotti
Starbucks® Grande Nonfat Caffè Latte

Calories: 270, Protein: 18g, Carbohydrate: 39g, Fat: 5g

**Snack** _____ or _____ **Quick Fix Snack**

1 T. peanut butter on 5 low-fat whole-wheat
crackers

Calories: 170, Protein: 14g, Carbohydrate: 8g, Fat: 9g

1 package (6) crackers with peanut butter

Calories: 329, Protein: 6g, Carbohydrate: 21g, Fat: 9g

**Lunch** _____ or _____ **Quick Fix Lunch**

Salad of: 1 oz. lean ham, 1 oz. provolone
cheese, 1 egg, hard-boiled, sliced, and
2 c. mixed vegetables with 2 T. low-fat
salad dressing
½ c. natural applesauce

Calories: 310, Protein: 25g, Carbohydrate: 23g, Fat: 13g

Starkist® Lunch To-Go
8–10 baby carrots
1 piece of fruit

Calories: 329, Protein: 20g, Carbohydrate: 42g, Fat: 9g

**Snack** _____

Kashi GoLean Roll!® Chocolate Peanut bar
or similar bar

Calories: 190, Protein: 12g, Carbohydrate: 28g, Fat: 5g

**Dinner** _____ or _____ **Quick Fix Dinner**

6 oz. grilled lean steak
1½ c. grilled onions, mushrooms, and
broccoli
1 small sweet potato with 1 T. light margarine

Calories: 697, Protein: 65g, Carbohydrate: 37g, Fat: 31g

*Frozen*
Stouffer's® Skillets Broccoli & Beef
V8® 100% vegetable juice (8 oz.)

Calories: 380, Protein: 22g, Carbohydrate: 56g, Fat: 7g

or

*Restaurant*
Applebee's® Restaurant Tortilla Chicken
Wrap

Calories: 480, Protein: 28g, Carbohydrate: 62g, Fat: 13g

**Snack/Dessert** _____

6 oz. light yogurt
1 T. low-fat granola

Calories: 150, Protein: 13g, Carbohydrate: 23g, Fat: 1g

# WEEK ONE, DAY TWO

**Breakfast** _____ or _____ **Quick Fix Breakfast**

2 T. chopped walnuts

1 c. cantaloupe

1 c. low-fat cottage cheese

Calories: 315, Protein: 34g, Carbohydrate: 23g, Fat: 9g

Breakstone's® Cottage Doubles (cottage cheese with fruit)

1 oz. almonds (about 23)

Calories: 304, Protein: 20g, Carbohydrate: 20g, Fat: 16g

**Snack** _____ or _____ **Quick Fix Snack**

1 c. nonfat milk

10 almonds

1 c. berries

Calories: 222, Protein: 12g, Carbohydrate: 35g, Fat: 6g

1 Keribar™ Cherry Almond

Calories: 160, Protein: 6g, Carbohydrate: 22g, Fat: 7g

**Lunch** _____ or _____ **Quick Fix Lunch**

3 oz. turkey breast with ½ oz. shredded cheese in a small whole-wheat pita

1½ c. mixed vegetable salad with 2 T. low-fat salad dressing

½ c. cooked green beans

15 red grapes

Calories: 325, Protein: 30g, Carbohydrate: 40g, Fat: 5g

Lean Cuisine® Mandarin Chicken

Calories: 270, Protein: 14g, Carbohydrate: 46g, Fat: 4g

**Snack** _____

1 oz. string cheese with 100-calorie serving of whole-wheat crackers

Calories: 164, Protein: 8g, Carbohydrate: 15g, Fat: 8g

**Dinner** _____ or _____ **Quick Fix Dinner**

8 oz. shrimp mixed with 1½ c. stir fry vegetables and 2 T. light margarine

1 c. cooked brown rice

Calories: 601, Protein: 59g, Carbohydrate: 61g, Fat: 13g

*Frozen*

Stouffer's® Grilled Chicken Teriyaki

1 c. raw vegetables

Calories: 325, Protein: 23g, Carbohydrate: 55g, Fat: 4g

or

*Restaurant*

P F Chang's® Lemon Pepper Shrimp

Calories: 520, Protein: 44g, Carbohydrate: 31g, Fat: 25g

**Snack/Dessert** _____

The Skinny Cow® Low-Fat Ice Cream Sandwich (chocolate or vanilla)

Calories: 140, Protein: 3g, Carbohydrate: 30g, Fat: 2g

# WEEK ONE, DAY THREE

**Breakfast** _____ or _____ **Quick Fix Breakfast**

2 eggs or ½ c. egg substitute, scrambled
  with ½ c. mushrooms
½ small whole-wheat bagel with butter spray
1 c. nonfat milk

Calories: 302, Protein: 22g, Carbohydrate: 31g, Fat: 10g

McDonald's® Egg McMuffin

Calories: 300, Protein: 17g, Carbohydrate: 30g, Fat: 12g

**Snack** _____ or _____ **Quick Fix Snack**

1 oz. peanuts
1 c. sliced kiwi

Calories: 222, Protein: 8g, Carbohydrate: 19g, Fat: 12g

2 Yoplait® Go-Gurt or other portable yogurt

Calories: 160, Protein: 4g, Carbohydrate: 26g, Fat: 4g

**Lunch** _____ or _____ **Quick Fix Lunch**

Salad of: 3 oz. tuna (water-packed) with 1 T.
  light mayonnaise, 3 c. mixed greens, and
  5 cherry tomatoes with 2 T. low-fat salad
  dressing and 1 T. sunflower seeds
1 medium apple

Calories: 313, Protein: 25g, Carbohydrate: 29g, Fat: 11g

Wendy's® Mandarin Chicken Salad with
  1 packet of low-fat dressing (without
  noodles)

Calories: 410, Protein: 27g, Carbohydrate: 43g, Fat: 16g

**Snack** _____

6 pieces of sushi (California roll)

Calories: 160, Protein: 23g, Carbohydrate: 10g, Fat: 3g

**Dinner** _____ or _____ **Quick Fix Dinner**

6 oz. baked chicken
½ c. steamed broccoli and ½ c. steamed
  carrots mixed with 2 T. light margarine
1 c. cooked whole-wheat pasta

Calories: 593, Protein: 54g, Carbohydrate: 50g, Fat: 19g

*Frozen*

Stouffer's® Skillets Chicken & Pasta
1 oz. Parmesan cheese

Calories: 440, Protein: 37g, Carbohydrate: 42g, Fat: 14g

or

*Restaurant*

Panera Bread® You Pick Two: 1 c. Low-Fat
  Chicken Noodle Soup and ½ Grilled Chicken
  Caesar Salad with 2 T. dressing
1 slice of sourdough bread

Calories: 434, Protein: 19g, Carbohydrate: 49g, Fat: 18g

**Snack/Dessert** _____

1 oz. low-fat mozzarella cheese
1 medium apple

Calories: 150, Protein: 9g, Carbohydrate: 14g, Fat: 5g

# WEEK ONE, DAY FOUR

**Breakfast** _____ or _____ **Quick Fix Breakfast**

2 eggs, hard-boiled or ½ c. egg substitute, scrambled

1 slice whole-grain toast with low-sugar jelly

½ c. low-fat vanilla yogurt

Calories: 322, Protein: 21g, Carbohydrate: 44g, Fat: 11g

Kashi® GoLean Roll! Chocolate Peanut Bar or similar bar

Starbucks® Grande Nonfat Cappuccino

Calories: 290, Protein: 21g, Carbohydrate: 42g, Fat: 5g

**Snack** _____ or _____ **Quick Fix Snack**

2 oz. tuna (water-packed) on 5 whole-wheat crackers

1 medium pear

Calories: 206, Protein: 15g, Carbohydrate: 27g, Fat: 4g

1 c. Campbell's® Select Gold Label Soup, Blended Red Pepper Black Bean

3 low-sodium saltine crackers

Calories: 159, Protein: 4g, Carbohydrate: 29g, Fat: 3g

**Lunch** _____ or _____ **Quick Fix Lunch**

3 oz. grilled 90% lean hamburger

1 c. assorted raw vegetables with 2 T. low-fat yogurt veggie dip

1 c. mixed berries

Calories: 318, Protein: 26g, Carbohydrate: 26g, Fat: 11g

Wendy's® Small Chili

Side salad with 1 packet of low-fat dressing

Calories: 365, Protein: 18g, Carbohydrate: 52g, Fat: 9g

**Snack** _____

½ c. (dry measure) oatmeal

Calories: 150, Protein: 5g, Carbohydrate: 27g, Fat: 3g

**Dinner** _____ or _____ **Quick Fix Dinner**

6 oz. lean baked pork chop

1½ c. mixed vegetable salad and ½ c. cauliflower with 2 T. low-fat salad dressing

Small whole-grain roll

Calories: 626, Protein: 55g, Carbohydrate: 45g, Fat: 24g

*Frozen*

Stouffer's® Beef Pot Roast

½ c. natural applesauce

½ c. low-fat cottage cheese

Calories: 400, Protein: 30g, Carbohydrate: 47g, Fat: 11g

or

*Restaurant*

Olive Garden® Chicken Giardino (lunch portion)

Dinner salad with 1 T. Italian dressing on the side

Calories: 451, Protein: 26g, Carbohydrate: 41g, Fat: 16g

**Snack/Dessert** _____

1 oz. mixed nuts

Calories: 168, Protein: 5g, Carbohydrate: 7g, Fat: 14g

## WEEK ONE, DAY FIVE

**Breakfast** _____ or _____ **Quick Fix Breakfast**

3 oz. lean ham

½ whole-wheat English muffin

½ c. melon

1 c. nonfat milk

Calories: 337, Protein: 31g, Carbohydrate: 39g, Fat: 6g

Burger King® Croissan'wich with Egg
(no cheese)

Calories: 260, Protein: 10g, Carbohydrate: 25g, Fat: 13g

**Snack** _____ or _____ **Quick Fix Snack**

1 oz. low-fat mozzarella cheese

2 rice cakes

1 c. strawberries

Calories: 206, Protein: 9g, Carbohydrate: 27g, Fat: 5g

McDonald's® Yogurt Parfait

Calories: 160, Protein: 4g, Carbohydrate: 31g, Fat: 2g

**Lunch** _____ or _____ **Quick Fix Lunch**

3 oz. crab or imitation crab meat (water-
packed) with 1 T. light mayonnaise in small
whole-wheat pita

1 c. vegetable soup

1 cucumber with 2 T. low-fat salad dressing

Calories: 322, Protein: 25g, Carbohydrate: 24g, Fat: 14g

2 Taco Bell® Fresco Style Grilled Steak
Soft Tacos

Calories: 340, Protein: 22g, Carbohydrate: 42g, Fat: 10g

**Snack** _____

1 T. peanut butter

1 medium apple

Calories: 160, Protein: 4g, Carbohydrate: 19g, Fat: 8g

**Dinner** _____ or _____ **Quick Fix Dinner**

6 oz. baked white fish

1½ c. steamed zucchini, onions, and red and
green pepper with 1 T. light margarine

1 small sweet potato with 1 T. light margarine

Calories: 602, Protein: 52g, Carbohydrate: 42g, Fat: 25g

*Frozen*

Stouffer's® Grilled Herb Chicken

1 c. baby carrots with 2 T. low-fat dressing

Calories: 351, Protein: 21g, Carbohydrate: 42g, Fat: 11g

or

*Restaurant*

Subway® 12-inch Turkey Breast on Wheat with
all the vegetables (no mayonnaise, no cheese)

Calories: 560, Protein: 36g, Carbohydrate: 92g, Fat: 9g

**Snack/Dessert** _____

So Delicious™ Dairy Free, Sugar Free Fudge Bar

½ c. sliced mangos

Calories: 134, Protein: 2g, Carbohydrate: 26g, Fat: 5g

# WEEK ONE, DAY SIX

**Breakfast** _____ or _____ **Quick Fix Breakfast**

Power shake: Mix 1 scoop whey protein
powder, 1 c. blueberries, ½ c. low-fat
berry yogurt, and ½ c. nonfat milk

Calories: 345, Protein: 35g, Carbohydrate: 44g, Fat: 1g

Yoplait® Nouriche Drink (11 oz.)

Calories: 260, Protein: 10g, Carbohydrate: 55g, Fat: 0g

**Snack** _____ or _____ **Quick Fix Snack**

½ c. low-fat cottage cheese
1 c. sliced peaches

Calories: 201, Protein: 14g, Carbohydrate: 32g, Fat: 2g

1 apple
10 almonds

Calories: 129, Protein: 4g, Carbohydrate: 17g, Fat: 6g

**Lunch** _____ or _____ **Quick Fix Lunch**

Salad of: 6 oz. salmon (water-packed), 1 c.
assorted raw vegetables and 1½ c. mixed
greens with 2 T. low-fat salad dressing
15 grapes

Calories: 304, Protein: 32g, Carbohydrate: 26g, Fat: 8g

Burger King® Tendergrill Chicken Sandwich
(without ½ the bun)

Calories: 325, Protein: 33g, Carbohydrate: 29g, Fat: 8g

**Snack** _____

6 oz. low-fat yogurt
1 T. low-fat granola

Calories: 150, Protein: 13g, Carbohydrate: 24g, Fat: 1g

**Dinner** _____ or _____ **Quick Fix Dinner**

6 oz. roasted white meat turkey
1½ c. cooked green beans with 1 T. light
margarine
1 small baked potato with 1 T. light
margarine

Calories: 599, Protein: 57g, Carbohydrate: 63g, Fat: 17g

*Frozen*

Stouffer's® Skillets Steak Teriyaki

Calories: 310, Protein: 17g, Carbohydrate: 49g, Fat: 5g

or

*Restaurant*

Boston Market® ¼ White Original Rotisserie
Chicken, no skin
4.8 oz. steamed vegetables
5½ oz. garlic dill new potatoes

Calories: 440, Protein: 46g, Carbohydrate: 36g, Fat: 13g

**Snack/Dessert** _____

2 oz. tuna (water-packed) with 1 t. light
mayonnaise
5 celery stalks

Calories: 147, Protein: 15g, Carbohydrate: 1g, Fat: 8g

# WEEK ONE, DAY SEVEN

**Breakfast** _____ or _____ **Quick Fix Breakfast**

3 oz. smoked salmon on ½ small whole-
wheat bagel with 2 T. low-fat cream cheese
½ c. strawberries

Calories: 312, Protein: 24g, Carbohydrate: 34g, Fat: 10g

1¼ c. Kashi® GoLean High Protein &
High Fiber Cereal
1 c. nonfat milk

Calories: 265, Protein: 24g, Carbohydrate: 49g, Fat: 1g

**Snack** _____ or _____ **Quick Fix Snack**

1 egg, hard-boiled
6 low-sodium saltine crackers
1 medium apple

Calories: 220, Protein: 9g, Carbohydrate: 30g, Fat: 7g

1½ oz. tropical trail mix

Calories: 171, Protein: 3g, Carbohydrate: 28g, Fat: 7g

**Lunch** _____ or _____ **Quick Fix Lunch**

Salad of: 3 oz. turkey breast, 2 c. mixed greens
and assorted vegetables, and ½ c. dried
cranberries with 2 T. low-fat salad dressing

Calories: 347, Protein: 33g, Carbohydrate: 38g, Fat: 7g

Arby's® Regular Roast Beef

Calories: 320, Protein: 20g, Carbohydrate: 34g, Fat: 13g

**Snack** _____

Starbucks® Grande Nonfat Caffè Latte with
sugar-free vanilla flavoring

Calories: 160, Protein: 16g, Carbohydrate: 24g, Fat: 0g

**Dinner** _____ or _____ **Quick Fix Dinner**

6 oz. grilled chicken
1½ c. mixed greens with 2 T. low-fat salad
dressing
½ c. steamed broccoli
1 c. cooked brown rice

Calories: 585, Protein: 58g, Carbohydrate: 49g, Fat: 18g

*Frozen*

Stouffer's® Skillets Garlic Chicken
¼ c. slivered almonds

Calories: 500, Protein: 31g, Carbohydrate: 48g, Fat: 21g

or

*Restaurant*

Chinese Restaurant, Chicken Stir Fry

Calories: 531, Protein: 47g, Carbohydrate: 61g, Fat: 11g

**Snack/Dessert** _____

The Skinny Cow® Low-Fat Ice Cream
Sandwich (chocolate or vanilla)

Calories: 140, Protein: 3g, Carbohydrate: 30g, Fat: 2g

# WEEK TWO, DAY ONE

**Breakfast** _____ or _____ **Quick Fix Breakfast**

2 slices whole-wheat toast with 2 slices
melted low-fat mozzarella cheese

4 to 6 slices tomato

Calories: 300, Protein: 18g, Carbohydrate: 40g, Fat: 8g

Myoplex® Lite Ready-to-Drink Shake or
similar product

1 small banana

Calories: 280, Protein: 26g, Carbohydrate: 43g, Fat: 3g

**Snack** _____ or _____ **Quick Fix Snack**

2 oz. tuna (water-packed) on 5 whole-wheat
crackers

1 medium apple

Calories: 206, Protein: 15g, Carbohydrate: 27g, Fat: 4g

1 package (6) crackers with peanut butter

Calories: 200, Protein: 6g, Carbohydrate: 21g, Fat: 9g

**Lunch** _____ or _____ **Quick Fix Lunch**

Salad of: 3 oz. lean ham, 1 egg, hard-boiled,
sliced, 1 T. slivered almonds, and 2 c. mixed
vegetables with 2 T. low-fat salad dressing

1 medium pear

Calories: 301, Protein: 29g, Carbohydrate: 21g, Fat: 11g

Weight Watchers® Smart Ones Creamy
Parmesan Chicken

Piece of fruit

Calories: 270, Protein: 23g, Carbohydrate: 27g, Fat: 8g

**Snack** _____

1 c. nonfat milk blended with ½ c. frozen
berries and sugar-free sweetener

Calories: 140, Protein: 8g, Carbohydrate: 27g, Fat: 0g

**Dinner** _____ or _____ **Quick Fix Dinner**

6 oz. grilled low-fat turkey sausage

1 c. grilled onions and peppers

1 c. green beans sautéed in 1 T. olive oil

1 medium French bread roll

Calories: 585, Protein: 42g, Carbohydrate: 52g, Fat: 23g

*Frozen*

Stouffer's® Grilled Lemon Pepper Chicken

¼ c. slivered almonds

Small whole-wheat roll

Piece of fruit

Calories: 515, Protein: 30g, Carbohydrate: 47g, Fat: 23g

or

*Restaurant*

Red Lobster® Light-House Menu King Crab Legs

1 side of seasoned fresh broccoli

Calories: 546, Protein: 106g, Carbohydrate: 10g, Fat: 9g

**Snack/Dessert** _____

1 packet Nestlé® Rich Chocolate Hot Cocoa
Mix made with 1 c. nonfat milk

Calories: 171, Protein: 9g, Carbohydrate: 27g, Fat: 3g

# WEEK TWO, DAY TWO

**Breakfast** _____ or _____ **Quick Fix Breakfast**

2 eggs or ½ c. egg substitute, scrambled
with ½ c. mushrooms

½ small whole-wheat bagel with butter spray

1 c. nonfat milk

Calories: 302, Protein: 22g, Carbohydrate: 31g, Fat: 10g

Breakstone's® Cottage Doubles (cottage
cheese with fruit)

1 oz. almonds (about 23)

Calories: 304, Protein: 20g, Carbohydrate: 20g, Fat: 16g

**Snack** _____ or _____ **Quick Fix Snack**

1 T. peanut butter on 8 low-fat whole-wheat
crackers

Calories: 205, Protein: 15g, Carbohydrate: 13g, Fat: 10g

Odwalla® Super Protein Original Vitamin
Fruit Juice Drink

Calories: 190, Protein: 10g, Carbohydrate: 35g, Fat: 1g

**Lunch** _____ or _____ **Quick Fix Lunch**

3 oz. chicken breast cubed with ½ oz.
shredded cheese wrapped in a small
whole-wheat tortilla

2 c. tomato, onion, cucumber, and cooked
green beans mixed with 2 T. low-fat Italian
dressing

½ c. sliced peaches

Calories: 325, Protein: 30g, Carbohydrate: 40g, Fat: 5g

McDonald's® Caesar Salad with Grilled
Chicken with 2 T. low-fat dressing

Calories: 260, Protein: 30g, Carbohydrate: 12g, Fat: 9g

**Snack** _____

Starbucks® Grande Nonfat Caffè Latte with
sugar-free hazelnut flavoring

Calories: 160, Protein: 16g, Carbohydrate: 24g, Fat: 0g

**Dinner** _____ or _____ **Quick Fix Dinner**

4 oz. grilled 90% lean ground beef hamburger
on a whole-wheat bun

1½ c. baby carrots with 2 T. low-fat dip

Calories: 542, Protein: 35g, Carbohydrate: 60g, Fat: 18g

*Frozen*

Stouffer's® Single-Serving Lasagna with
Meat and Sauce

2 cans Del Monte® Lite Mixed Fruit (4 oz. each)

Calories: 450, Protein: 24g, Carbohydrate: 64g, Fat: 11g

or

*Restaurant*

P F Chang's® Lemon Pepper Shrimp

Calories: 520, Protein: 44g, Carbohydrate: 31g, Fat: 25g

**Snack/Dessert** _____

3 low-fat chocolate chip cookies

Calories: 135, Protein: 2g, Carbohydrate: 22g, Fat: 5g

# WEEK TWO, DAY THREE

**Breakfast** _____ or _____ **Quick Fix Breakfast**

3 oz. lean ham
½ whole-wheat English muffin
½ c. melon
1 c. nonfat milk

Calories: 337, Protein: 31g, Carbohydrate: 39g, Fat: 6g

Myoplex® Lite Ready-to-Drink Shake or
  similar product
1 small banana

Calories: 280, Protein: 26g, Carbohydrate: 43g, Fat: 3g

**Snack** _____ or _____ **Quick Fix Snack**

1 oz. low-fat mozzarella cheese on 2 rice cakes
1 c. blueberries

Calories: 206, Protein: 9g, Carbohydrate: 27g, Fat: 5g

2 Yoplait® Go-Gurt or other portable yogurt

Calories: 160, Protein: 4g, Carbohydrate: 26g, Fat: 4g

**Lunch** _____ or _____ **Quick Fix Lunch**

Salad of: 3 oz. tuna (water-packed) with 1 T.
  light mayonnaise, mixed with ½ c. sliced
  grapes and 1 T. chopped walnuts on top
  of 3 c. mixed greens and ½ c. shredded
  carrots with 2 T. low-fat salad dressing

Calories: 315, Protein: 25g, Carbohydrate: 24g, Fat: 13g

Stouffer's® Chicken a la King

Calories: 370, Protein: 20g, Carbohydrate: 45g, Fat: 12g

**Snack** _____

1 T. peanut butter
1 medium apple

Calories: 160, Protein: 4g, Carbohydrate: 19g, Fat: 8g

**Dinner** _____ or _____ **Quick Fix Dinner**

Omelet made with 3 eggs or ¾ c. egg
  substitute and 1 oz. low-fat cheese
1 c. fresh steamed broccoli with 1 T. light
  margarine
2 slices whole-wheat toast with 1 T. light
  margarine

Calories: 572, Protein: 40g, Carbohydrate: 49g, Fat: 24g

*Frozen*
Stouffer's® Grilled Chicken Portabello
½ c. natural applesauce
Small whole-wheat roll

Calories: 330, Protein: 20g, Carbohydrate: 48g, Fat: 6g
or
*Restaurant*
Panera Bread® You Pick Two: 1 c. Low-Fat
  Chicken Noodle Soup and ½ Grilled
  Chicken Caesar Salad with 2 T. dressing
1 slice of sourdough bread

Calories: 434, Protein: 19g, Carbohydrate: 49g, Fat: 18g

**Snack/Dessert** _____

6 oz. light yogurt
1 T. low-fat granola

Calories: 150, Protein: 13g, Carbohydrate: 23g, Fat: 1g

# WEEK TWO, DAY FOUR

**Breakfast** _____ or _____ **Quick Fix Breakfast**

Power shake: Mix 1 scoop whey protein
powder, 1 c. pineapple, ½ c. low-fat
yogurt, and 1 c. nonfat milk

Calories: 325, Protein: 35g, Carbohydrate: 43g, Fat: 1g

Larabar® Apple Pie Bar or similar bar
Starbucks® Grande Nonfat Cappuccino

Calories: 290, Protein: 13g, Carbohydrate: 37g, Fat: 9g

**Snack** _____ or _____ **Quick Fix Snack**

1 oz. peanuts
1 c. sliced peaches

Calories: 222, Protein: 8g, Carbohydrate: 19g, Fat: 12g

1 c.Campbell's® Select Gold Label Soup,
Blended Red Pepper Black Bean
3 low-sodium saltine crackers

Calories: 159, Protein: 4g, Carbohydrate: 29g, Fat: 3g

**Lunch** _____ or _____ **Quick Fix Lunch**

3 oz. lean roast beef
6 oz. vegetable juice
1½ c. mixed vegetable salad with 2 T. low-
fat yogurt veggie dip
1 c. mixed berries

Calories: 318, Protein: 26g, Carbohydrate: 26g, Fat: 11g

Burger King® Fire-Grilled Burger
Piece of fruit

Calories: 350, Protein: 15g, Carbohydrate: 45g, Fat: 12g

**Snack** _____

1 oz. string cheese with 100-calorie serving
of whole-wheat crackers

Calories: 164, Protein: 8g, Carbohydrate: 15g, Fat: 8g

**Dinner** _____ or _____ **Quick Fix Dinner**

6 oz. grilled chicken brushed with 2 T. BBQ
sauce
2 c. mixed vegetable salad and ½ oz. shredded
cheese with 2 T. low-fat salad dressing
Small whole-wheat roll

Calories: 577, Protein: 58g, Carbohydrate: 34g, Fat: 21g

*Frozen*
Stouffer's® Skillets Steak Teriyaki
1 medium apple
1 oz. low-fat cheese

Calories: 430, Protein: 25g, Carbohydrate: 60g, Fat: 10g

or

*Restaurant*
Subway® 12-inch Roast Beef on Wheat with
all the vegetables (no mayonnaise, no cheese)

Calories: 580, Protein: 38g, Carbohydrate: 90g, Fat: 10g

**Snack/Dessert** _____

½ c. fat-free sorbet
1 T. low-fat granola

Calories: 160, Protein: 1g, Carbohydrate: 37g, Fat: 1g

# WEEK TWO, DAY FIVE

### Breakfast _____ or _____ Quick Fix Breakfast

3 oz. smoked salmon on ½ small whole-wheat
  bagel with 2 T. low-fat cream cheese
½ c. strawberries

Calories: 312, Protein: 24g, Carbohydrate: 34g, Fat: 10g

Denny's® Fit Fair™ Veggie Omelette with
  English Muffin (dry)

Calories: 330, Protein: 25g, Carbohydrate: 37g, Fat: 8g

### Snack _____ or _____ Quick Fix Snack

1 egg, hard-boiled
6 low-sodium saltine crackers
1 medium pear

Calories: 220, Protein: 9g, Carbohydrate: 30g, Fat: 7g

½ whole-grain bagel
1 T. light cream cheese

Calories: 155, Protein: 7g, Carbohydrate: 27g, Fat: 3g

### Lunch _____ or _____ Quick Fix Lunch

3 oz. cooked shredded chicken mixed with
  1 T. light mayonnaise and 1 T. pickle relish
  in a small whole-wheat pita
1 c. vegetable soup
1 cucumber, sliced with 1 T. low-fat salad
  dressing

Calories: 322, Protein: 25g, Carbohydrate: 24g, Fat: 14g

Quiznos® Sierra Smoked Turkey (Lite Selection,
  no cheese) with Raspberry-Chipotle Sauce

Calories: 350, Protein: 23g, Carbohydrate: 53g, Fat: 6g

### Snack _____

1 packet Quaker® Instant Oatmeal, Lower
  Sugar Apples & Cinnamon
1 medium nectarine

Calories: 172, Protein: 5g, Carbohydrate: 37g, Fat: 2g

### Dinner _____ or _____ Quick Fix Dinner

6 oz. baked cod with lemon pepper
1½ c. steamed asparagus tossed with 1 t.
  olive oil and ½ t. chopped garlic
1 medium baked potato with 2 T. light
  margarine

Calories: 584, Protein: 50g, Carbohydrate: 49g, Fat: 20g

***Frozen***

Stouffer's® Grilled Herb Chicken
1 c. baby carrots with 2 T. low-fat dressing

Calories: 351, Protein: 21g, Carbohydrate: 42g, Fat: 11g

or

***Restaurant***

Chinese Restaurant, Chicken Stir Fry

Calories: 531, Protein: 47g, Carbohydrate: 61g, Fat: 11g

### Snack/Dessert _____

½ c. low-fat cottage cheese
½ c. pears

Calories: 141, Protein: 14g, Carbohydrate: 18g, Fat: 2g

# WEEK TWO, DAY SIX

**Breakfast** _____ or _____ **Quick Fix Breakfast**

Power shake: Mix 1 scoop whey protein powder, 1 c. blueberries, ½ c. low-fat berry yogurt, and ½ c. nonfat milk

Calories: 345, Protein: 35g, Carbohydrate: 44g, Fat: 1g

Jamba Juice® Protein Berry Pizzazz (452g serving)

Calories: 280, Protein: 15g, Carbohydrate: 56g, Fat: 1g

**Snack** _____ or _____ **Quick Fix Snack**

1 c. nonfat milk
10 almonds
1 c. strawberries

Calories: 222, Protein: 12g, Carbohydrate: 35g, Fat: 6g

1 apple
10 almonds

Calories: 129, Protein: 4g, Carbohydrate: 17g, Fat: 6g

**Lunch** _____ or _____ **Quick Fix Lunch**

6 oz. crab or imitation crab (water-packed)
1 c. assorted raw vegetables and 1½ c. mixed greens with 2 T. low-fat salad dressing
15 grapes

Calories: 304, Protein: 32g, Carbohydrate: 26g, Fat: 8g

Arby's® Regular Roast Beef

Calories: 320, Protein: 20g, Carbohydrate: 34g, Fat: 13g

**Snack** _____

½ c. (dry measure) oatmeal

Calories: 150, Protein: 5g, Carbohydrate: 27g, Fat: 3g

**Dinner** _____ or _____ **Quick Fix Dinner**

6 oz. baked Italian marinated chicken (marinate in low-fat Italian dressing for 30–60 min.)
1½ c. cooked green beans with ½ T. light margarine and 1 T. slivered almonds
1 small baked sweet potato with ½ T. light margarine

Calories: 590, Protein: 57g, Carbohydrate: 63g, Fat: 16g

*Frozen*
Stouffer's® Beef Pot Roast
½ c. sliced peaches
6 oz. light yogurt

Calories: 360, Protein: 23g, Carbohydrate: 49g, Fat: 8g

or

*Restaurant*
Boston Market® ¼ White Original Rotisserie Chicken, no skin
4.8 oz. steamed vegetables
5½ oz. garlic dill new potatoes

Calories: 440, Protein: 46g, Carbohydrate: 36g, Fat: 13g

**Snack/Dessert** _____

1 oz. low-fat cheese
1 medium apple

Calories: 137, Protein: 8g, Carbohydrate: 15g, Fat: 5g

# WEEK TWO, DAY SEVEN

**Breakfast** _____ or _____ **Quick Fix Breakfast**

½ c. (dry measure) oatmeal with 2 T. wheat germ and ¼ c. raisins

Calories: 308, Protein: 10g, Carbohydrate: 62g, Fat: 4g

Odwalla® Super Protein Original Vitamin Fruit Juice Drink

1 frozen whole-grain waffle with 1 T. peanut butter

Calories: 356, Protein: 16g, Carbohydrate: 53g, Fat: 10g

**Snack** _____ or _____ **Quick Fix Snack**

½ c. low-fat cottage cheese

1 c. sliced pineapple

Calories: 201, Protein: 14g, Carbohydrate: 32g, Fat: 2g

1 package (6) crackers with peanut butter

Calories: 200, Protein: 6g, Carbohydrate: 21g, Fat: 9g

**Lunch** _____ or _____ **Quick Fix Lunch**

Salad of: 3 oz. grilled chicken breast, 1½ c. mixed vegetables, and ¼ c. dried cranberries with 1 T. low-fat salad dressing

6 oz. vegetable juice

Calories: 347, Protein: 33g, Carbohydrate: 38g, Fat: 7g

Chinese Restaurant, Chicken and Broccoli

Calories: 300, Protein: 31g, Carbohydrate: 19g, Fat: 9g

**Snack** _____

Low-fat whole-grain nutrition bar

Red Bull® Energy Drink, sugar free

Calories: 150, Protein: 5g, Carbohydrate: 26g, Fat: 2g

**Dinner** _____ or _____ **Quick Fix Dinner**

6 oz. grilled turkey tenderloin

1½ c. mixed greens with 2 T. low-fat salad dressing

½ c. steamed cauliflower

1 c. cooked brown rice with 1 T. light margarine

Calories: 590, Protein: 58g, Carbohydrate: 41g, Fat: 19g

*Frozen*

Stouffer's® Skillets Garlic Chicken

¼ c. slivered almonds

Calories: 500, Protein: 31g, Carbohydrate: 48g, Fat: 21g

or

*Restaurant*

Subway® 12-inch Turkey Breast on Wheat with all the vegetables (no mayonnaise, no cheese)

Calories: 560, Protein: 36g, Carbohydrate: 92g, Fat: 9g

**Snack/Dessert** _____

1 oz. low-fat mozzarella cheese

5 low-fat whole-wheat crackers

Calories: 150, Protein: 9g, Carbohydrate: 14g, Fat: 5g

## WEEK THREE, DAY ONE

**Breakfast** _____ or _____ **Quick Fix Breakfast**

2 eggs or ½ c. egg substitute, scrambled
    with ½ c. chopped red and green peppers
½ whole-wheat English muffin with butter spray
1 c. nonfat milk

Calories: 302, Protein: 22g, Carbohydrate: 31g, Fat: 10g

Myoplex® Lite Ready-to-Drink Shake or
    or similar product
1 small banana

Calories: 280, Protein: 26g, Carbohydrate: 43g, Fat: 3g

**Snack** _____ or _____ **Quick Fix Snack**

½ c. low-fat cottage cheese
1 c. sliced peaches

Calories: 201, Protein: 14g, Carbohydrate: 32g, Fat: 2g

Odwalla® Nourishing Food Bar, Carrot

Calories: 220, Protein: 4g, Carbohydrate: 43g, Fat: 4g

**Lunch** _____ or _____ **Quick Fix Lunch**

Salad of: 3 oz. turkey, 1 oz. low-fat crumbled
    feta cheese, 1 T. slivered almonds, 2 c.
    mixed vegetables and greens with 2 T.
    low-fat salad dressing
1 medium apple

Calories: 310, Protein: 29g, Carbohydrate: 21g, Fat: 12g

Weight Watchers® Smart Ones Chicken
    Oriental
Piece of fruit

Calories: 290, Protein: 12g, Carbohydrate: 42g, Fat: 8g

**Snack** _____

Starbucks® Grande Nonfat Caffè Latte with
    sugar-free vanilla flavoring

Calories: 160, Protein: 16g, Carbohydrate: 24g, Fat: 0g

**Dinner** _____ or _____ **Quick Fix Dinner**

5 oz. grilled London Broil
1 c. onions and mushrooms sautéed in 2 t.
    olive oil
⅔ c. rice pilaf

Calories: 526, Protein: 51g, Carbohydrate: 38g, Fat: 20g

*Frozen*
Stouffer's® Stuffed Peppers (2)
Small whole-wheat roll with 1 T. light margarine

Calories: 463, Protein: 16g, Carbohydrate: 57g, Fat: 19g

or

*Restaurant*
Red Lobster® Light-House Menu Grilled
    Jumbo Shrimp Dinner
Garden salad with 2 T. vingarette red wine
    dressing
1 Cheddar Bay® biscuit

Calories: 404, Protein: 31g, Carbohydrate: 32g, Fat: 17g

**Snack/Dessert** _____

1 oz. roasted almonds

Calories: 150, Protein: 8g, Carbohydrate: 4g, Fat: 12g

# WEEK THREE, DAY TWO

**Breakfast** _____ or _____ **Quick Fix Breakfast**

½ c. (dry measure) oatmeal with 2 T. wheat
germ and ¼ c. dried blueberries

Calories: 308, Protein: 10g, Carbohydrate: 62g, Fat: 4g

Starbucks® Biscotti
Starbucks® Grande Nonfat Caffè Latte

Calories: 270, Protein: 18g, Carbohydrate: 39g, Fat: 5g

**Snack** _____ or _____ **Quick Fix Snack**

1 T. peanut butter on 8 low-fat whole-wheat
crackers

Calories: 205, Protein: 15g, Carbohydrate: 13g, Fat: 10g

1 package (6) crackers with peanut butter

Calories: 200, Protein: 6g, Carbohydrate: 21g, Fat: 9g

**Lunch** _____ or _____ **Quick Fix Lunch**

3 oz. lean roast beef with ½ oz. shredded
mozzarella cheese wrapped in a small
whole-wheat tortilla

2 c. tomato, cucumber, onion, and red pepper
with 2 T. low-fat Italian dressing

½ c. sliced strawberries

Calories: 325, Protein: 30g, Carbohydrate: 40g, Fat: 5g

Burger King® Veggie Burger (no mayonnaise,
no cheese)

Calories: 340, Protein: 23g, Carbohydrate: 46g, Fat: 8g

**Snack** _____

1 oz. cheese with 100-calorie serving of
whole-wheat crackers

Calories: 164, Protein: 8g, Carbohydrate: 15g, Fat: 8g

**Dinner** _____ or _____ **Quick Fix Dinner**

5 oz. cooked lean taco-seasoned ground beef
with 1 oz. low-fat cheese; 1 c. chopped
tomatoes, onions, and shredded lettuce; and
½ c. salsa all wrapped in a whole-wheat
tortilla with 1 T. low-fat sour cream

Calories: 495, Protein: 47g, Carbohydrate: 48g, Fat: 13g

*Frozen*
Stouffer's® Turkey Tetrazzini
1 c. steamed asparagus
½ c. sliced peaches

Calories: 480, Protein: 22g, Carbohydrate: 57g, Fat: 18g

or

*Restaurant*
Ruby Tuesday® Creole Catch
Dinner salad with 2 T. light dressing
Fresh steamed broccoli (hold the butter sauce)

Calories: 517, Protein: 42g, Carbohydrate: 29g, Fat: 26g

**Snack/Dessert** _____

1 chocolate Tofutti Cuties® Sandwich

Calories: 130, Protein: 2g, Carbohydrate: 16g, Fat: 5g

# WEEK THREE, DAY THREE

**Breakfast** _____ or _____ **Quick Fix Breakfast**

2 T. chopped walnuts

1 c. cantaloupe

1 c. low-fat cottage cheese

Calories: 315, Protein: 34g, Carbohydrate: 23g, Fat: 9g

Subway® 6-inch Honey Mustard Ham and
Egg Breakfast Sandwich

Calories: 310, Protein: 20g, Carbohydrate: 50g, Fat: 5g

**Snack** _____ or _____ **Quick Fix Snack**

1 oz. peanuts

1 c. sliced kiwi fruit

Calories: 222, Protein: 8g, Carbohydrate: 19g, Fat: 12g

McDonald's® Vanilla Reduced-Fat Ice Cream
Cone

Calories: 150, Protein: 4g, Carbohydrate: 24g, Fat: 4g

**Lunch** _____ or _____ **Quick Fix Lunch**

Salad of: 3 oz. white meat chicken with 1 T.
light mayonnaise, mixed with ½ c. sliced
grapes and 1 T. chopped walnuts on top of
3 c. mixed greens with 2 T. low-fat salad
dressing

1 medium peach

Calories: 319, Protein: 25g, Carbohydrate: 25g, Fat: 13g

Taco Bell® Fresco Style Fiesta Burrito
Chicken

Calories: 340, Protein: 16g, Carbohydrate: 50g, Fat: 8g

**Snack** _____

Nature Valley® Oats 'n Honey Granola Bars
(1 pouch containing 2 bars)

Calories: 180, Protein: 4g, Carbohydrate: 29g, Fat: 6g

**Dinner** _____ or _____ **Quick Fix Dinner**

6 oz. chicken baked with 1 c. marinara
sauce

2 c. whole-wheat pasta

1 T. fresh grated Parmesan cheese

1 c. fresh steamed broccoli

Calories: 515, Protein: 50g, Carbohydrate: 60g, Fat: 8g

*Frozen*

Stouffer's® Chicken a la King

1 c. steamed broccoli

Small whole-wheat roll

Calories: 480, Protein: 27g, Carbohydrate: 66g, Fat: 12g

or

*Restaurant*

Panera Bread® Vegetarian Roasted Red
Pepper and Lentil Soup with California
Mission Chicken Salad

Calories: 530, Protein: 32g, Carbohydrate: 48g, Fat: 23g

**Snack/Dessert** _____

6 oz. light yogurt

1 T. low-fat granola

Calories: 150, Protein: 13g, Carbohydrate: 23g, Fat: 1g

# WEEK THREE, DAY FOUR

**Breakfast** _____ or _____ **Quick Fix Breakfast**

2 slices whole-wheat toast with 2 slices melted low-fat mozzarella cheese

4 to 6 slices tomato

Calories: 300, Protein: 18g, Carbohydrate: 40g, Fat: 8g

Clif Nectar® Cranberry, Apricot, & Almond Bar

Starbucks® Grande Nonfat Cappuccino

Calories: 270, Protein: 12g, Carbohydrate: 43g, Fat: 6g

**Snack** _____ or _____ **Quick Fix Snack**

1 c. nonfat milk

10 almonds

1 c. berries

Calories: 222, Protein: 12g, Carbohydrate: 35g, Fat: 6g

1 c. Campbell's® Select Gold Label Soup, Blended Red Pepper Black Bean

3 low-sodium saltine crackers

Calories: 159, Protein: 4g, Carbohydrate: 29g, Fat: 3g

**Lunch** _____ or _____ **Quick Fix Lunch**

3 oz. lean ham with mustard on whole-wheat bun

6 oz. vegetable juice

1½ c. mixed vegetable salad with 2 T. low-fat yogurt veggie dip

1 medium apple

Calories: 318, Protein: 26g, Carbohydrate: 26g, Fat: 11g

Panda Express® Kung Pao Chicken

Calories: 240, Protein: 16g, Carbohydrate: 12g, Fat: 15g

**Snack** _____

½ c. low-fat cottage cheese

1 can Del Monte® Lite Mixed Fruit (4 oz.)

Calories: 150, Protein: 14g, Carbohydrate: 19g, Fat: 3g

**Dinner** _____ or _____ **Quick Fix Dinner**

6 oz. grilled lean pork

2 c. mixed vegetable salad with 2 T. low-fat salad dressing

Small whole-grain roll

Calories: 527, Protein: 55g, Carbohydrate: 34g, Fat: 19g

*Frozen*

Stouffer's® Single-Serving Lasagna with Meat and Sauce

Small salad with 2 T. low-fat dressing

Calories: 435, Protein: 26g, Carbohydrate: 53g, Fat: 13g

or

*Restaurant*

Carrabba's Italian Grill® Chicken Bryan with vegetable and dinner salad with 2 T. light dressing

Calories: 497, Protein: 58g, Carbohydrate: 10g, Fat: 25g

**Snack/Dessert** _____

1 oz. dry roasted peanuts

Calories: 160, Protein: 5g, Carbohydrate: 7g, Fat: 13g

# WEEK THREE, DAY FIVE

**Breakfast** _____ or _____ **Quick Fix Breakfast**

2 eggs, hard-boiled or ½ c. egg substitute, scrambled

1 slice whole-grain toast with low-sugar jelly

½ c. low-fat vanilla yogurt

Calories: 322, Protein: 21g, Carbohydrate: 44g, Fat: 11g

Burger King® Croissan'wich with Egg (no cheese)

Calories: 260, Protein: 10g, Carbohydrate: 25g, Fat: 13g

**Snack** _____ or _____ **Quick Fix Snack**

2 oz. tuna (water-packed) on 5 whole-wheat crackers

1 medium pear

Calories: 206, Protein: 15g, Carbohydrate: 27g, Fat: 4g

Odwalla® Super Protein Original Vitamin Fruit Juice Drink

Calories: 190, Protein: 10g, Carbohydrate: 35g, Fat: 1g

**Lunch** _____ or _____ **Quick Fix Lunch**

3 oz. lean roast beef in a small whole-wheat pita with 2 tomato slices, ½ c. shredded lettuce, and 1 T. low-fat salad dressing

1 pickle

1 c. vegetable soup

Calories: 326, Protein: 26g, Carbohydrate: 24g, Fat: 14g

Quiznos® Honey Bourbon Chicken on Wheat Bread (Lite Selection)

Calories: 359, Protein: 29g, Carbohydrate: 45g, Fat: 7g

**Snack** _____

1 T. peanut butter

1 medium apple

Calories: 160, Protein: 4g, Carbohydrate: 19g, Fat: 8g

**Dinner** _____ or _____ **Quick Fix Dinner**

1 c. chicken chili with beans and 1 oz. low-fat cheese

1 c. cooked green beans with 1 T. light margarine

⅔ c. cooked brown rice

Calories: 529, Protein: 36g, Carbohydrate: 62g, Fat: 15g

*Frozen*

Stouffer's® Grilled Lemon Pepper Chicken

1 c. baby carrots with 2 T. low-fat dressing

Small whole-grain roll

Calories: 435, Protein: 27g, Carbohydrate: 55g, Fat: 12g

or

*Restaurant*

Olive Garden® Shrimp Primavera (½ dinner portion)

Dinner salad with dressing on the side (use 2 T.)

Calories: 553, Protein: 26g, Carbohydrate: 65g, Fat: 21g

**Snack/Dessert** _____

½ c. low-fat cottage cheese

1 c. cantaloupe

Calories: 154, Protein: 15g, Carbohydrate: 19g, Fat: 2g

# WEEK THREE, DAY SIX

## Breakfast _____ or _____ **Quick Fix Breakfast**

3 oz. lean ham
½ whole-wheat English muffin
½ c. pineapple
1 c. nonfat milk

Calories: 315, Protein: 34g, Carbohydrate: 23g, Fat: 9g

Yoplait® Nouriche Drink (11 oz.)

Calories: 260, Protein: 10g, Carbohydrate: 55g, Fat: 0g

## Snack _____ or _____ **Quick Fix Snack**

1 oz. low-fat mozzarella cheese
2 rice cakes
1 c. strawberries

Calories: 206, Protein: 9g, Carbohydrate: 27g, Fat: 5g

1 apple
10 almonds
1 packet Nestlé® Rich Chocolate Hot Cocoa
  Mix (add hot water)

Calories: 209, Protein: 4g, Carbohydrate: 32g, Fat: 9g

## Lunch _____ or _____ **Quick Fix Lunch**

Salad of: 3 oz. grilled chicken breast, 1 c.
  assorted raw vegetables, 1½ c. mixed greens,
  and ¼ c. dried cranberries with 2 T. low-fat
  salad dressing

Calories: 315, Protein: 32g, Carbohydrate: 29g, Fat: 8g

Blimpie® Turkey Italiano Panini

Calories: 390, Protein: 22g, Carbohydrate: 45g, Fat: 10g

## Snack _____

1 c. nonfat milk blended with ½ c. frozen
  berries and sugar-free sweetner

Calories: 140, Protein: 8g, Carbohydrate: 27g, Fat: 0g

## Dinner _____ or _____ **Quick Fix Dinner**

6 oz. boiled or grilled shrimp
1 c. angel hair pasta with 1 T. light margarine
1½ c. cooked spinach with 1 T. light
  margarine
½ c. sliced fruit

Calories: 478, Protein: 35g, Carbohydrate: 62g, Fat: 10g

*Frozen*
Stouffer's® Skillets Garlic Chicken
1 c. cooked green beans
1 apple, sliced

Calories: 446, Protein: 30g, Carbohydrate: 68g, Fat: 6g

or

*Restaurant*
Boston Market® Roasted Sirloin (5 oz.)
4.7 oz. green beans
5½ oz. garlic dill new potatoes

Calories: 530, Protein: 43g, Carbohydrate: 36g, Fat: 23g

## Snack/Dessert _____

1 oz. low-fat cheese
1 medium apple

Calories: 137, Protein: 8g, Carbohydrate: 15g, Fat: 5g

## WEEK THREE, DAY SEVEN

**Breakfast** _____ or _____ **Quick Fix Breakfast**

Power shake: Mix 1 scoop whey protein
powder, 1 c. blueberries, ½ c. low-fat berry
yogurt, and ½ c. nonfat milk

Calories: 345, Protein: 35g, Carbohydrate: 44g, Fat: 1g

1¼ c. Kashi® GoLean High Protein & High
Fiber Cereal
1 c. nonfat milk

Calories: 280, Protein: 17g, Carbohydrate: 48g, Fat: 3g

**Snack** _____ or _____ **Quick Fix Snack**

1 egg, hard-boiled
6 low-sodium saltine crackers
1 medium apple

Calories: 220, Protein: 9g, Carbohydrate: 30g, Fat: 7g

½ whole-grain bagel with 1 T. light cream
cheese

Calories: 155, Protein: 7g, Carbohydrate: 27g, Fat: 3g

**Lunch** _____ or _____ **Quick Fix Lunch**

3 oz. tuna (water-packed) with 1 T. light
mayonnaise wrapped in a small whole-
wheat tortilla
2 c. assorted raw vegetables with 2 T. fat-free
ranch dip

Calories: 316, Protein: 31g, Carbohydrate: 30g, Fat: 8g

Jamba Juice® Pizza Protein Stick
1 large orange

Calories: 316, Protein: 11g, Carbohydrate: 55g, Fat: 6g

**Snack** _____

Nature Valley® Oats 'n Honey Granola Bars
(1 pouch containing 2 bars)

Calories: 180, Protein: 4g, Carbohydrate: 29g, Fat: 6g

**Dinner** _____ or _____ **Quick Fix Dinner**

6 oz. grilled or baked salmon
1½ c. mixed greens with 2 T. low-fat salad
dressing
½ c. cole slaw
⅔ c. cooked brown rice

Calories: 504, Protein: 46g, Carbohydrate: 44g, Fat: 16g

*Frozen*

Stouffer's® Beef Pot Roast
½ c. natural applesauce
1 c. steamed cauliflower with 1 T. light
margarine

Calories: 401, Protein: 20g, Carbohydrate: 51g, Fat: 13g

or

*Restaurant*

Chinese Restaurant, Chicken and Broccoli

Calories: 580, Protein: 42g, Carbohydrate: 62g, Fat: 18g

**Snack/Dessert** _____

1 McDonald's® Oatmeal Raisin Cookie

Calories: 140, Protein: 2g, Carbohydrate: 22g, Fat: 5g

## WEEK FOUR, DAY ONE

**Breakfast** _____ or _____ **Quick Fix Breakfast**

3 oz. lean ham

1 slice whole-wheat bread

½ c. melon

1 c. nonfat milk

Calories: 337, Protein: 31g, Carbohydrate: 39g, Fat: 6g

Myoplex® Lite Ready-to-Drink Shake or
similar product

1 large peach

Calories: 251, Protein: 26g, Carbohydrate: 35g, Fat: 3g

**Snack** _____ or _____ **Quick Fix Snack**

1 c. nonfat milk

10 almonds

1 c. strawberries

Calories: 222, Protein: 12g, Carbohydrate: 35g, Fat: 6g

Luna® Bar, Iced Oatmeal Raisin

Calories: 180, Protein: 10g, Carbohydrate: 28g, Fat: 4g

**Lunch** _____ or _____ **Quick Fix Lunch**

3 oz. lean roast beef with 1 oz. low-fat
Swiss cheese in a small whole-wheat pita

2 c. raw vegetables with 2 T. low-fat dip

1 small apple

Calories: 361, Protein: 29g, Carbohydrate: 36g, Fat: 11g

Taco Bell® Bean Burrito with mild sauce
(no cheese or sour cream)

1 medium apple

Calories: 370, Protein: 17g, Carbohydrate: 52g, Fat: 10g

**Snack** _____

1 c. nonfat milk blended with ½ c. frozen
berries and sugar-free sweetener

Calories: 140, Protein: 8g, Carbohydrate: 27g, Fat: 0g

**Dinner** _____ or _____ **Quick Fix Dinner**

6 oz. grilled fresh fish

2 c. zucchini, onions, mushrooms, and
red peppers, grilled in 1 T. olive oil

1 medium baked potato

Calories: 585, Protein: 42g, Carbohydrate: 52g, Fat: 23g

*Frozen*

Stouffer's® Grilled Herb Chicken

1 c. baby carrots with ¼ c. slivered almonds
and 2 T. low-fat dressing

Calories: 531, Protein: 28g, Carbohydrate: 47g, Fat: 26g

or

*Restaurant*

Carrabba's Italian Grill® house salad (dressing
on the side)

Chicken Gratella without grill baste

1 slice Italian bread without butter

Calories: 480, Protein: 54g, Carbohydrate: 20g, Fat: 19g

**Snack/Dessert** _____

1 oz. roasted almonds

Calories: 150, Protein: 8g, Carbohydrate: 4g, Fat: 12g

## WEEK FOUR, DAY TWO

**Breakfast** _____ or _____ **Quick Fix Breakfast**

2 T. chopped walnuts

1 c. cantaloupe

1 c. low-fat cottage cheese

Calories: 315, Protein: 34g, Carbohydrate: 23g, Fat: 9g

Breakstone's® Cottage Doubles (cottage cheese with fruit)

1 oz. almonds (about 23)

Calories: 304, Protein: 20g, Carbohydrate: 20g, Fat: 16g

**Snack** _____ or _____ **Quick Fix Snack**

1 oz. peanuts

1 c. sliced kiwi fruit

Calories: 222, Protein: 8g, Carbohydrate: 19g, Fat: 12g

½ whole grain bagel with 1 T. light cream cheese

Calories: 155, Protein: 7g, Carbohydrate: 27g, Fat: 3g

**Lunch** _____ or _____ **Quick Fix Lunch**

3 oz. salmon (water-packed) tossed with 2 c. tomato, cucumber, onion, and cooked green beans, mixed with 2 T. low-fat Italian salad dressing

½ c. blueberries

½ c. strawberries

Calories: 334, Protein: 30g, Carbohydrate: 40g, Fat: 6g

McDonald's® Premium Grilled Chicken Classic Sandwich (no mayonnaise)

Calories: 370, Protein: 32g, Carbohydrate: 51g, Fat: 5g

**Snack** _____

Low-fat whole-grain nutrition bar

Calories: 140, Protein: 5g, Carbohydrate: 23g, Fat: 2g

**Dinner** _____ or _____ **Quick Fix Dinner**

Omelet made with 3 eggs or ¾ c. egg substitute and 1 oz. low-fat cheese

1 c. fresh steamed green beans with 1 T. light margarine

2 slices whole-wheat toast with 1 T. light margarine

Calories: 572, Protein: 40g, Carbohydrate: 49g, Fat: 24g

*Frozen*

Lean Cuisine® French Bread Cheese Pizza

Frozen Vegetable Medley cooked with ½ T. olive oil

Calories: 460, Protein: 20g, Carbohydrate: 60g, Fat: 14g

or

*Restaurant*

Ruby Tuesday® Turkey Burger Wrap

Small house salad with 2 T. low-fat dressing

Calories: 470, Protein: 48g, Carbohydrate: 15g, Fat: 24g

**Snack/Dessert** _____

The Skinny Cow® Low-Fat Ice Cream Sandwich (vanilla or chocolate)

Calories: 140, Protein: 3g, Carbohydrate: 30g, Fat: 2g

# WEEK FOUR, DAY THREE

**Breakfast** _____ or _____ **Quick Fix Breakfast**

2 eggs or ½ c. egg substitute, scrambled
   with ½ c. mushrooms
½ small whole-wheat bagel with butter spray
1 c. nonfat milk

Calories: 302, Protein: 22g, Carbohydrate: 31g, Fat: 10g

McDonald's® Egg McMuffin

Calories: 300, Protein: 17g, Carbohydrate: 30g, Fat: 12g

**Snack** _____ or _____ **Quick Fix Snack**

1 T. peanut butter on 8 low-fat whole-wheat
   crackers

Calories: 205, Protein: 15g, Carbohydrate: 13g, Fat: 10g

2 Yoplait® Go-Gurt or other portable yogurt

Calories: 160, Protein: 4g, Carbohydrate: 26g, Fat: 4g

**Lunch** _____ or _____ **Quick Fix Lunch**

3 oz. cooked shredded chicken mixed with
   1 T. light mayonnaise and 1 T. pickle
   relish in a whole-wheat roll
1 c. vegetable soup
10 baby carrots

Calories: 322, Protein: 25g, Carbohydrate: 24g, Fat: 14g

Quiznos® Turkey Lite on Wheat Bread
   (Lite Selection)

Calories: 334, Protein: 24g, Carbohydrate: 52g, Fat: 6g

**Snack** _____

6 oz. low-fat yogurt
1 T. low-fat granola

Calories: 150, Protein: 13g, Carbohydrate: 24g, Fat: 1g

**Dinner** _____ or _____ **Quick Fix Dinner**

6 oz. grilled chicken brushed with 2 T.
   BBQ sauce
1 c. mixed vegetable salad and ½ oz. shredded
   cheese with 1 T. low-fat dressing
1 ear corn (grilled) with 1 T. light margarine
1 c. cubed melon

Calories: 563, Protein: 58g, Carbohydrate: 43g, Fat: 18g

*Frozen*

Lean Cuisine® Sesame Chicken
1½ c. nonfat milk

Calories: 469, Protein: 28g, Carbohydrate: 67g, Fat: 10g

or

*Restaurant*

Panera Bread® You Pick Two: ½ Mediterranean
   Veggie Sandwich and Low-Fat Vegetarian
   Black Bean Soup

Calories: 455, Protein: 21g, Carbohydrate: 81g, Fat: 7g

**Snack/Dessert** _____

½ c. fat-free sorbet
1 T. low-fat granola

Calories: 160, Protein: 1g, Carbohydrate: 37g, Fat: 1g

# WEEK FOUR, DAY FOUR

## Breakfast     or     Quick Fix Breakfast

Power shake: Mix 1 scoop whey protein
   powder, 1 small banana, ½ c. low-fat
   yogurt, and 1 c. nonfat milk

Calories: 325, Protein: 35g, Carbohydrate: 43g, Fat: 1g

Kashi® GoLean Roll! Chocolate Peanut Bar
   or similar bar
Starbucks® Grande Nonfat Cappuccino

Calories: 290, Protein: 21g, Carbohydrate: 42g, Fat: 5g

## Snack     or     Quick Fix Snack

2 oz. tuna (water-packed) on 5 whole-wheat
   crackers
1 medium orange

Calories: 206, Protein: 15g, Carbohydrate: 27g, Fat: 4g

1 c. Campbell's® Select Gold Label Soup,
   Blended Red Pepper Black Bean
3 low-sodium saltine crackers

Calories: 159, Protein: 4g, Carbohydrate: 29g, Fat: 3g

## Lunch     or     Quick Fix Lunch

Salad of: 2 oz. lean ham, 1 egg, hard-boiled,
   sliced, 1 oz. low-fat cheese, and 2½ c. mixed
   vegetables with 2 T. low-fat salad dressing
1 medium apple

Calories: 348, Protein: 34g, Carbohydrate: 26g, Fat: 12g

Arby's® Regular Roast Beef

Calories: 320, Protein: 20g, Carbohydrate: 34g, Fat: 13g

## Snack

1 oz. cheese with 100-calorie serving of
   whole-wheat crackers

Calories: 164, Protein: 8g, Carbohydrate: 15g, Fat: 8g

## Dinner     or     Quick Fix Dinner

6 oz. baked orange roughy fish brushed with
   1 t. olive oil and ½ t. chopped garlic
2 c. steamed carrots, broccoli, and
   cauliflower with 1 T. light margarine
1 medium baked potato with 1 T. light
   margarine

Calories: 584, Protein: 50g, Carbohydrate: 49g, Fat: 20g

*Frozen*
Lean Cuisine® Teriyaki Steak Bowl
1 c. baby carrots

Calories: 330, Protein: 22g, Carbohydrate: 47g, Fat: 6g

or

*Restaurant*
Boston Market® ¼ White Original Rotisserie
   Chicken, no skin
4.8 oz. steamed vegetables
5½ oz. garlic dill new potatoes

Calories: 440, Protein: 46g, Carbohydrate: 36g, Fat: 13g

## Snack/Dessert

6 oz. light yogurt
1 T. low-fat granola

Calories: 150, Protein: 13g, Carbohydrate: 23g, Fat: 1g

# WEEK FOUR, DAY FIVE

**Breakfast** _____ or _____ **Quick Fix Breakfast**

3 oz. smoked salmon on ½ small whole-wheat
    bagel with 2 T. low-fat cream cheese
½ c. pineapple

Calories: 312, Protein: 24g, Carbohydrate: 34g, Fat: 10g

Burger King® Crossan'wich with Egg
    (no cheese)

Calories: 260, Protein: 10g, Carbohydrate: 25g, Fat: 13g

**Snack** _____ or _____ **Quick Fix Snack**

1 oz. low-fat mozzarella cheese
2 rice cakes
1 c. strawberries

Calories: 206, Protein: 9g, Carbohydrate: 27g, Fat: 5g

McDonald's® Yogurt Parfait

Calories: 160, Protein: 4g, Carbohydrate: 31g, Fat: 2g

**Lunch** _____ or _____ **Quick Fix Lunch**

Salad of: 3 oz. white meat chicken with 1 T.
    light mayonnaise, mixed with ¼ c. dried
    cranberries and 1 T. chopped walnuts on
    top of 3 c. mixed greens, and ½ c. shredded
    carrots with 2 T. low-fat salad dressing

Calories: 315, Protein: 25g, Carbohydrate: 24g, Fat: 13g

Wendy's® Caesar Chicken Salad with
    reduced-fat ranch dressing and garlic
    croutons

Calories: 350, Protein: 30g, Carbohydrate: 25g, Fat: 16g

**Snack** _____

1 packet Quaker® Instant Oatmeal, Lower
    Sugar Apples & Cinnamon
½ c. raspberries

Calories: 142, Protein: 4g, Carbohydrate: 29g, Fat: 2g

**Dinner** _____ or _____ **Quick Fix Dinner**

4 oz. grilled petite fillet
1 c. fresh steamed asparagus
½ c. pickled beets
1 small sweet potato with 1 T. light
    margarine

Calories: 580, Protein: 35g, Carbohydrate: 47g, Fat: 28g

*Frozen*
Lean Cuisine® Creamy Basil Chicken Bowl
1 c. raw vegetables

Calories: 336, Protein: 24g, Carbohydrate: 44g, Fat: 7g

or

*Restaurant*
Quiznos® Sierra Smoked Turkey (Lite Selection)
    with 1 slice of cheese and Raspberry-
    Chipotle Sauce

Calories: 458, Protein: 30g, Carbohydrate: 53g, Fat: 14g

**Snack/Dessert** _____

1 oz. low-fat cheese
1 medium apple

Calories: 137, Protein: 8g, Carbohydrate: 15g, Fat: 5g

# WEEK FOUR, DAY SIX

**Breakfast** _____ or _____ **Quick Fix Breakfast**

Power shake: Mix 1 scoop whey protein powder, 1 c. frozen raspberries, ½ c. low-fat berry yogurt, and ½ c. nonfat milk

Calories: 345, Protein: 35g, Carbohydrate: 44g, Fat: 1g

Yoplait® Nouriche Drink (11 oz.)

Calories: 260, Protein: 10g, Carbohydrate: 55g, Fat: 0g

**Snack** _____ or _____ **Quick Fix Snack**

½ c. low-fat cottage cheese
1 c. cubed melon

Calories: 201, Protein: 14g, Carbohydrate: 32g, Fat: 2g

1 apple
10 almonds

Calories: 129, Protein: 4g, Carbohydrate: 17g, Fat: 6g

**Lunch** _____ or _____ **Quick Fix Lunch**

6 oz. crab or imitation crab (water-packed) mixed with 2 T. low-fat ranch dressing and 1 T. chopped celery and onion wrapped in small whole-wheat tortilla
2 c. raw vegetables
15 grapes

Calories: 364, Protein: 34g, Carbohydrate: 37g, Fat: 9g

McDonald's® Cheeseburger
1 medium apple

Calories: 370, Protein: 15g, Carbohydrate: 50g, Fat: 12g

**Snack** _____

1 small banana
1 c. light yogurt

Calories: 165, Protein: 7g, Carbohydrate: 32g, Fat: 1g

**Dinner** _____ or _____ **Quick Fix Dinner**

6 oz. baked Italian marinated chicken (marinate in low-fat Italian dressing for 30–60 min.)
1½ c. cooked green beans with 1 T. light margarine and 1 T. slivered almonds
1 c. whole-wheat pasta

Calories: 590, Protein: 57g, Carbohydrate: 63g, Fat: 16g

*Frozen*

Lean Cuisine® Classic Five Cheese Lasagna
Frozen Vegetable Medley cooked with 1 T. light margarine

Calories: 420, Protein: 21g, Carbohydrate: 54g, Fat: 13g

or

*Restaurant*

Chinese Restaurant, Seafood and Vegetable Stir Fry

Calories: 527, Protein: 43g, Carbohydrate: 61g, Fat: 11g

**Snack/Dessert** _____

½ c. low-fat cottage cheese
½ c. pears

Calories: 141, Protein: 14g, Carbohydrate: 18g, Fat: 1g

# WEEK FOUR, DAY SEVEN

**Breakfast** _____ or _____ **Quick Fix Breakfast**

½ c. (dry measure) oatmeal with 2 T. wheat germ and ¼ c. raisins

Calories: 308, Protein: 10g, Carbohydrate: 62g, Fat: 4g

Myoplex® Lite Ready-to-Drink Shake or similar product

¾ c. fresh blueberries

Calories: 275, Protein: 25g, Carbohydrate: 40g, Fat: 2g

**Snack** _____ or _____ **Quick Fix Snack**

1 egg, hard-boiled

6 low-sodium saltine crackers

1 medium pear

Calories: 220, Protein: 9g, Carbohydrate: 30g, Fat: 7g

1 package (6) crackers with peanut butter

Red Bull® Energy Drink, sugar free

Calories: 210, Protein: 6g, Carbohydrate: 23g, Fat: 9g

**Lunch** _____ or _____ **Quick Fix Lunch**

3 oz. lean roast beef with 2 slices lettuce, tomato, onion, and 2 T. light mayonnaise on 2 slices light whole-wheat bread

1 c. vegetable soup

1 small banana

Calories: 347, Protein: 29g, Carbohydrate: 34g, Fat: 9g

Wendy's® Fish Sandwich with ketchup (omit the tartar sauce)

Calories: 360, Protein: 17g, Carbohydrate: 52g, Fat: 10g

**Snack** _____

1 packet Nestlé® Rich Chocolate Hot Cocoa Mix (add hot water)

½ Clif Nectar® Cranberry, Apricot, & Almond Bar

Calories: 165, Protein: 2g, Carbohydrate: 30g, Fat: 6g

**Dinner** _____ or _____ **Quick Fix Dinner**

5 oz. grilled pork tenderloin

1½ c. mixed greens with 2 T. low-fat salad dressing

½ c. steamed cauliflower

1 c. cooked brown rice with 1 T. light margarine

Calories: 590, Protein: 58g, Carbohydrate: 41g, Fat: 19g

*Frozen*

Lean Cuisine® Steak, Cheddar, and Mushroom Panini

1 Campbell's® Microwaveable Tomato Soup

Calories: 440, Protein: 23g, Carbohydrate: 67g, Fat: 9g

or

*Restaurant*

Chili's® Chicken Fajita Pita

Calories: 450, Protein: 43g, Carbohydrate: 35g, Fat: 17g

**Snack/Dessert** _____

1 oz. low-fat mozzarella cheese

5 low-fat whole-wheat crackers

Calories: 150, Protein: 9g, Carbohydrate: 14g, Fat: 5g

# WEEK FIVE, DAY ONE

**Breakfast** _____ or _____ **Quick Fix Breakfast**

Power shake: Mix 1 scoop whey protein powder, 1 c. strawberries, ½ c. low-fat vanilla yogurt, and 1 c. nonfat milk

Calories: 325, Protein: 35g, Carbohydrate: 43g, Fat: 1g

Breakstone's® Cottage Doubles (cottage cheese with fruit)

1 oz. almonds (about 23)

Calories: 304, Protein: 20g, Carbohydrate: 20g, Fat: 16g

**Snack** _____ or _____ **Quick Fix Snack**

1 c. nonfat milk

10 roasted almonds

1 c. strawberries

Calories: 222, Protein: 12g, Carbohydrate: 35g, Fat: 6g

Cold Fusion® Protein Juice Bar

Calories: 130, Protein: 11g, Carbohydrate: 23g, Fat: 0g

**Lunch** _____ or _____ **Quick Fix Lunch**

Salad of: 1 oz. lean ham, 1 oz. turkey, 1 oz. low-fat cheese, 1 medium apple, diced, 3 c. mixed greens, and ½ c. chopped vegetables with 2 T. low-fat salad dressing and 1 T. sunflower seeds

Calories: 313, Protein: 25g, Carbohydrate: 29g, Fat: 11g

2 Taco Bell® Fresco Style Grilled Steak Soft Tacos

Calories: 340, Protein: 22g, Carbohydrate: 42g, Fat: 10g

**Snack** _____

Starbucks® Grande Nonfat Caffè Latte with sugar-free vanilla flavoring

Calories: 160, Protein: 16g, Carbohydrate: 24g, Fat: 0g

**Dinner** _____ or _____ **Quick Fix Dinner**

6 oz. grilled pork tenderloin

1½ c. carrots and snap peas, grilled in 1 T. light margarine

¾ c. cooked brown rice

Calories: 619, Protein: 48g, Carbohydrate: 55g, Fat: 23g

*Frozen*

Lean Cuisine® Balsamic-Glazed Chicken

Calories: 380, Protein: 18g, Carbohydrate: 60g, Fat: 7g

or

*Restaurant*

Olive Garden® Shrimp Primavera (½ dinner portion)

Dinner salad with dressing on the side (use 2 T.)

Calories: 553, Protein: 26g, Carbohydrate: 65g, Fat: 21g

**Snack/Dessert** _____

6 oz. light yogurt

1 T. low-fat granola

Calories: 150, Protein: 13g, Carbohydrate: 23g, Fat: 1g

# WEEK FIVE, DAY TWO

**Breakfast** _____ or _____ **Quick Fix Breakfast**

½ c. (dry measure) oatmeal with 2 T. wheat germ and ¼ c. raisins

Calories: 308, Protein: 10g, Carbohydrate: 62g, Fat: 4g

Myoplex® Lite Ready-to-Drink Shake or similar product

20 red grapes

Calories: 258, Protein: 26g, Carbohydrate: 38g, Fat: 3g

**Snack** _____ or _____ **Quick Fix Snack**

1 oz. low-fat mozzarella cheese

2 rice cakes

1 c. sliced peaches

Calories: 206, Protein: 9g, Carbohydrate: 27g, Fat: 5g

1 package (6) crackers with peanut butter

Calories: 200, Protein: 6g, Carbohydrate: 21g, Fat: 9g

**Lunch** _____ or _____ **Quick Fix Lunch**

3 oz. grilled 90% lean hamburger on a whole-wheat bun

1½ c. mixed vegetable salad with 2 T. low-fat salad dressing

½ c. sliced peaches

Calories: 326, Protein: 29g, Carbohydrate: 30g, Fat: 10g

Wendy's® Frescata Roasted Turkey Sandwich (without the basil pesto)

Calories: 350, Protein: 20g, Carbohydrate: 49g, Fat: 8g

**Snack** _____

1 oz. string cheese with 100-calorie serving of whole-wheat crackers

Calories: 164, Protein: 8g, Carbohydrate: 15g, Fat: 8g

**Dinner** _____ or _____ **Quick Fix Dinner**

6 oz. grilled chicken

2 c. steamed broccoli and cauliflower with 1 T. light margarine

3–4 small new skin potatoes with 1 T. light margarine

Calories: 477, Protein: 50g, Carbohydrate: 40g, Fat: 13g

*Frozen*

Lean Cuisine® Jumbo Rigatoni with Meatballs

1 oz. Parmesan cheese

Calories: 490, Protein: 32g, Carbohydrate: 57g, Fat: 15g

or

*Restaurant*

Boston Market® ¼ White Original Rotisserie Chicken, no skin

4.8 oz. steamed vegetables

5½ oz. garlic dill new potatoes

Calories: 440, Protein: 46g, Carbohydrate: 36g, Fat: 13g

**Snack/Dessert** _____

1 McDonald's® Oatmeal Raisin Cookie

Calories: 140, Protein: 2g, Carbohydrate: 22g, Fat: 5g

# WEEK FIVE, DAY THREE

**Breakfast** _____ or _____ **Quick Fix Breakfast**

3 oz. smoked salmon on ½ small whole-
  wheat bagel with 2 T. low-fat cream cheese
½ c. strawberries

Calories: 312, Protein: 24g, Carbohydrate: 34g, Fat: 10g

Subway® 6-inch Honey Mustard Ham and
  Egg Breakfast Sandwich

Calories: 310, Protein: 20g, Carbohydrate: 50g, Fat: 5g

**Snack** _____ or _____ **Quick Fix Snack**

1 egg, hard-boiled
6 low-sodium saltine crackers
1 medium apple

Calories: 220, Protein: 9g, Carbohydrate: 30g, Fat: 7g

2 Yoplait Go-Gurt® or other portable yogurt

Calories: 160, Protein: 4g, Carbohydrate: 26g, Fat: 4g

**Lunch** _____ or _____ **Quick Fix Lunch**

3 oz. tuna (water-packed) and 1 hard-boiled
  egg mixed with 1 T. low-fat mayonnaise
  on 2 slices light whole-wheat bread
1 c. steamed chilled green beans mixed
  with 1 T. low-fat dressing
½ c. natural applesauce

Calories: 343, Protein: 23g, Carbohydrate: 38g, Fat: 11g

McDonald's® Asian Salad with Grilled
  Chicken and low-fat sesame-ginger
  dressing

Calories: 380, Protein: 32g, Carbohydrate: 37g, Fat: 12g

**Snack** _____

McDonald's® Vanilla Reduced-Fat Ice
  Cream Cone

Calories: 150, Protein: 4g, Carbohydrate: 24g, Fat: 4g

**Dinner** _____ or _____ **Quick Fix Dinner**

2 c. lean chili made with 90% lean beef
  and pinto beans
1 c. cooked green beans
Small dinner salad with 1 T. low-fat salad
  dressing
6 low-sodium saltine crackers

Calories: 515, Protein: 40g, Carbohydrate: 55g, Fat: 15g

*Frozen*

Lean Cuisine® Steak Tips Dijon
Frozen Vegetable Medley cooked with ½ T.
  olive oil

Calories: 440, Protein: 21g, Carbohydrate: 54g, Fat: 15g

or

*Restaurant*

Red Lobster® Lighthouse Menu Rock Lobster
Baked potato (no butter)
Seasoned vegetables

Calories: 575, Protein: 64g, Carbohydrate: 45g, Fat: 15g

**Snack/Dessert** _____

1 oz. low-fat mozzarella cheese
1 medium apple

Calories: 150, Protein: 9g, Carbohydrate: 14g, Fat: 5g

# WEEK FIVE, DAY FOUR

**Breakfast** _____  or  _____ **Quick Fix Breakfast**

Power shake: Mix 1 scoop whey protein
   powder, 1 c. cantaloupe, ½ c. low-fat
   berry yogurt, and ½ c. nonfat milk

Calories: 345, Protein: 35g, Carbohydrate: 44g, Fat: 1g

Larabar® Apple Pie Bar
Starbucks® Grande Nonfat Cappuccino

Calories: 290, Protein: 13g, Carbohydrate: 37g, Fat: 9g

**Snack** _____  or  _____ **Quick Fix Snack**

½ c. low-fat cottage cheese
1 c. sliced peaches

Calories: 201, Protein: 14g, Carbohydrate: 32g, Fat: 2g

1 c. Campbell's® Select Gold Label Soup,
   Blended Red Pepper Black Bean
3 low-sodium saltine crackers

Calories: 159, Protein: 4g, Carbohydrate: 29g, Fat: 3g

**Lunch** _____  or  _____ **Quick Fix Lunch**

3 oz. grilled chicken breast
1 c. assorted raw vegetables with 2 T. low-fat
   dip
½ c. pickled beets
1 c. strawberries

Calories: 301, Protein: 23g, Carbohydrate: 35g, Fat: 6g

Lean Cuisine® Mandarin Chicken

Calories: 270, Protein: 14g, Carbohydrate: 46g, Fat: 4g

**Snack** _____

½ c. (dry measure) oatmeal

Calories: 150, Protein: 5g, Carbohydrate: 27g, Fat: 3g

**Dinner** _____  or  _____ **Quick Fix Dinner**

6 oz. marinated broiled flank steak
1½ c. sautéed cabbage, onions, and red
   and green pepper with 1 T. light margarine
1 small sweet potato with 1 T. light margarine

Calories: 626, Protein: 55g, Carbohydrate: 45g, Fat: 24g

*Frozen*

Lean Cuisine® Dinner-Time Selects Chicken
   Fettuccini

Calories: 390, Protein: 27g, Carbohydrate: 53g, Fat: 8g

or

*Restaurant*

Chinese Restaurant, Moo Shu Chicken

Calories: 430, Protein: 28g, Carbohydrate: 43g, Fat: 16g

**Snack/Dessert** _____

Eskimo Pie® Premium No Sugar Added
   Cookies & Cream Bar

Calories: 120, Protein: 2g, Carbohydrate: 17g, Fat: 7g

## WEEK FIVE, DAY FIVE

**Breakfast** _____    or    _____ **Quick Fix Breakfast**

2 slices whole-wheat toast with 2 slices
   melted low-fat mozzarella cheese
4 to 6 slices tomato

Calories: 300, Protein: 18g, Carbohydrate: 40g, Fat: 8g

Yoplait® Nouriche Drink (11 oz.)

Calories: 260, Protein: 10g, Carbohydrate: 55g, Fat: 0g

**Snack** _____    or    _____ **Quick Fix Snack**

2 oz. tuna (water-packed) on 5 whole-wheat
   crackers
1 medium pear

Calories: 206, Protein: 15g, Carbohydrate: 27g, Fat: 4g

McDonald's® Vanilla Reduced-Fat Ice-
   Cream Cone

Calories: 150, Protein: 4g, Carbohydrate: 24g, Fat: 4g

**Lunch** _____    or    _____ **Quick Fix Lunch**

3 oz. shrimp mixed with 1 T. light
   mayonnaise and 2 T. chopped celery and
   onion in small whole-wheat pita
1 c. vegetable soup with 1 sliced cucumber
½ c. fresh fruit

Calories: 302, Protein: 27g, Carbohydrate: 35g, Fat: 6g

Jamba Juice® Pizza Protein Stick
1 large orange

Calories: 316, Protein: 11g, Carbohydrate: 55g, Fat: 6g

**Snack** _____

1 T. peanut butter
1 medium apple

Calories: 160, Protein: 4g, Carbohydrate: 19g, Fat: 8g

**Dinner** _____    or    _____ **Quick Fix Dinner**

6 oz. baked white fish with 1 T. light
   margarine
1½ c. mixed greens with ½ c. cauliflower
Small whole-wheat roll with 1 T. light
   margarine

Calories: 602, Protein: 52g, Carbohydrate: 42g, Fat: 25g

*Frozen*

Lean Cuisine® Oven Roasted Beef Burgundy
V8® 100% vegetable juice (8 oz.)

Calories: 350, Protein: 19g, Carbohydrate: 53g, Fat: 7g

or

*Restaurant*

Panera Bread® You Pick Two: Tuscan
   Vegetable & Ditalini Soup and ½ Smokehouse
   Turkey Panini on Artisan Three Cheese Bread

Calories: 470, Protein: 29g, Carbohydrate: 55g, Fat: 15g

**Snack/Dessert** _____

½ c. low-fat cottage cheese
½ c. pears

Calories: 141, Protein: 14g, Carbohydrate: 18g, Fat: 1g

# WEEK FIVE, DAY SIX

**Breakfast** _____ or _____ **Quick Fix Breakfast**

2 eggs or ½ c. egg substitute, scrambled
with ½ c. mushrooms
½ small whole-wheat bagel with butter spray
1 c. nonfat milk

*Calories: 302, Protein: 22g, Carbohydrate: 31g, Fat: 10g*

Jamba Juice® Protein Berry Pizzazz
(452g serving)

*Calories: 280, Protein: 15g, Carbohydrate: 56g, Fat: 1g*

**Snack** _____ or _____ **Quick Fix Snack**

1 T. peanut butter on 8 low-fat whole-wheat
crackers

*Calories: 205, Protein: 15g, Carbohydrate: 13g, Fat: 10g*

1 apple
10 almonds

*Calories: 129, Protein: 4g, Carbohydrate: 17g, Fat: 6g*

**Lunch** _____ or _____ **Quick Fix Lunch**

Salad of: 6 oz. salmon (water-packed), 1 c.
assorted raw vegetables, 15 grapes, and
1½ c. mixed greens with 2 T. low-fat
salad dressing

*Calories: 304, Protein: 32g, Carbohydrate: 26g, Fat: 8g*

Starkist® Lunch To-Go
8–10 baby carrots
1 piece of fruit

*Calories: 329, Protein: 20g, Carbohydrate: 42g, Fat: 9g*

**Snack** _____

6 oz. low-fat yogurt
1 T. low-fat granola

*Calories: 150, Protein: 13g, Carbohydrate: 24g, Fat: 1g*

**Dinner** _____ or _____ **Quick Fix Dinner**

8 oz. crab or imitation crab (water-packed)
stir fried with 1½ c. stir fry vegetables,
cooking spray, and 1 T. light margarine
1 c. cooked brown rice with 1 T. light
margarine

*Calories: 601, Protein: 59g, Carbohydrate: 61g, Fat: 13g*

***Frozen***
Lean Cuisine® Margherita Pizza
½ c. low-fat cottage cheese

*Calories: 420, Protein: 28g, Carbohydrate: 54g, Fat: 12g*

or

***Restaurant***
Chili's® Chicken Fajita Pita

*Calories: 450, Protein: 43g, Carbohydrate: 35g, Fat: 17g*

**Snack/Dessert** _____

1 chocolate Tofutti Cuties® Sandwich

*Calories: 130, Protein: 2g, Carbohydrate: 16g, Fat: 5g*

# WEEK SIX, DAY TWO

**Breakfast** _____ or _____ **Quick Fix Breakfast**

2 T. chopped almonds

1 c. sliced melon

1 c. low-fat cottage cheese

Calories: 315, Protein: 34g, Carbohydrate: 23g, Fat: 9g

Jamba Juice® Protein Berry Pizzazz
(452g serving)

Calories: 280, Protein: 15g, Carbohydrate: 56g, Fat: 1g

**Snack** _____ or _____ **Quick Fix Snack**

1 c. nonfat milk

10 almonds

1 c. berries

Calories: 222, Protein: 12g, Carbohydrate: 35g, Fat: 6g

Odwalla® Super Protein Original Vitamin
Fruit Juice Drink

Calories: 190, Protein: 10g, Carbohydrate: 35g, Fat: 1g

**Lunch** _____ or _____ **Quick Fix Lunch**

3 oz. lean roast beef with 1 T. low-fat dip
on 2 slices light whole-grain bread

1 c. vegetable soup

15 red grapes

Calories: 386, Protein: 29g, Carbohydrate: 45g, Fat: 10g

Lean Cuisine® One-Dish Favorites
Chicken Fettuccini

Calories: 280, Protein: 21g, Carbohydrate: 33g, Fat: 7g

**Snack** _____

½ c. low-fat cottage cheese

1 can Del Monte® Lite Mixed Fruit (4 oz.)

Calories: 150, Protein: 14g, Carbohydrate: 19g, Fat: 3g

**Dinner** _____ or _____ **Quick Fix Dinner**

6 oz. grilled shrimp

1½ c. fresh steamed asparagus with 1 T.
light margarine

⅔ c. cooked brown rice with 1 T. light
margarine

Calories: 489, Protein: 49g, Carbohydrate: 44g, Fat: 13g

*Frozen*

Stouffer's® Grilled Chicken Portabello

½ c. sliced peaches

Small whole-wheat roll

Calories: 330, Protein: 20g, Carbohydrate: 48g, Fat: 6g

or

*Restaurant*

Fazoli's® Classic Pasta Ravioli with
Marinara Sauce

Calories: 600, Protein: 27g, Carbohydrate: 89g, Fat: 15g

**Snack/Dessert** _____

The Skinny Cow® Low-Fat Ice Cream
Sandwich (chocolate or vanilla)

Calories: 140, Protein: 3g, Carbohydrate: 30g, Fat: 2g

# WEEK SIX, DAY THREE

### Breakfast _____ or _____ Quick Fix Breakfast

½ c. (dry measure) oatmeal with 2 T. wheat germ and ¼ c. raisins

Calories: 308, Protein: 10g, Carbohydrate: 62g, Fat: 4g

McDonald's® Egg McMuffin

Calories: 300, Protein: 17g, Carbohydrate: 30g, Fat: 12g

### Snack _____ or _____ Quick Fix Snack

1 oz. peanuts

1 c. sliced kiwi fruit

Calories: 222, Protein: 8g, Carbohydrate: 19g, Fat: 12g

2 Yoplait® Go-Gurt or other portable yogurt

Calories: 160, Protein: 4g, Carbohydrate: 26g, Fat: 4g

### Lunch _____ or _____ Quick Fix Lunch

Salad of: 3 oz. tuna (water-packed), 1 c. assorted raw vegetables, and 1½ c. mixed greens with 2 T. low-fat salad dressing

1 orange

Calories: 304, Protein: 32g, Carbohydrate: 26g, Fat: 8g

Panda Express® Beef with Broccoli

1 Vegetable Spring Roll

Calories: 230, Protein: 13g, Carbohydrate: 22g, Fat: 10g

### Snack _____

1 T. peanut butter

1 medium apple

Calories: 160, Protein: 4g, Carbohydrate: 19g, Fat: 8g

### Dinner _____ or _____ Quick Fix Dinner

6 oz. grilled low-fat turkey sausage with red peppers and onions

1 c. steamed broccoli

1 medium boiled potato sautéed in 1 T. olive oil with garlic, salt, and pepper

Calories: 585, Protein: 42g, Carbohydrate: 52g, Fat: 23g

*Frozen*

Stouffer's® Skillets Garlic Chicken

1 medium apple

Calories: 380, Protein: 24g, Carbohydrate: 58g, Fat: 6g

or

*Restaurant*

Olive Garden® Chicken Marsala (½ dinner portion)

Dinner salad with dressing on the side (use 2 T.)

Calories: 552, Protein: 19g, Carbohydrate: 36g, Fat: 36g

### Snack/Dessert _____

6 oz. light yogurt

1 T. low-fat granola

Calories: 150, Protein: 13g, Carbohydrate: 23g, Fat: 1g

# WEEK SIX, DAY FOUR

**Breakfast** _____ or _____ **Quick Fix Breakfast**

3 oz. lean ham

½ whole-wheat English muffin

½ banana

1 c. nonfat milk

Calories: 337, Protein: 31g, Carbohydrate: 39g, Fat: 6g

Odwalla® Super Protein Original Vitamin
  Fruit Juice Drink

1 frozen whole-grain waffle with 1 T. peanut
  butter

Calories: 356, Protein: 16g, Carbohydrate: 53, Fat: 10g

**Snack** _____ or _____ **Quick Fix Snack**

2 oz. tuna (water-packed) on 5 whole-wheat
  crackers

1 medium apple

Calories: 206, Protein: 15g, Carbohydrate: 27g, Fat: 4g

1 c. Campbell's® Select Gold Label Soup,
  Blended Red Pepper Black Bean

3 low-sodium saltine crackers

Calories: 159, Protein: 5g, Carbohydrate: 26g, Fat: 4g

**Lunch** _____ or _____ **Quick Fix Lunch**

Grilled cheese made with 3 oz. low-fat
  cheese, 2 slices light whole-wheat bread,
  and 1 T. light margarine

1 c. tomato soup

Calories: 337, Protein: 26g, Carbohydrate: 38g, Fat: 9g

Stouffer's® Grilled Chicken Portabello

Calories: 210, Protein: 16g, Carbohydrate: 23g, Fat: 6g

**Snack** _____

1 oz. string cheese with 100-calorie serving
  of whole-wheat crackers

Calories: 164, Protein: 8g, Carbohydrate: 15g, Fat: 8g

**Dinner** _____ or _____ **Quick Fix Dinner**

Mexican omelet made with 3 eggs or ¾ c.
  egg substitute, 1 oz. low-fat cheese,
  ½ c. salsa, and 1 T. light margarine

2 slices whole-wheat toast with 1 T. light
  margarine

Calories: 471, Protein: 34g, Carbohydrate: 23g, Fat: 27g

*Frozen*

Stouffer's® Single-Serving Lasagne with Meat
  and Sauce

Frozen Vegetable Medley cooked with ½ T.
  olive oil

Calories: 470, Protein: 26g, Carbohydrate: 48g, Fat: 18g

or

*Restaurant*

Subway® 12-inch Turkey Breast on Wheat with
  all the vegetables (no mayonnaise, no cheese)

Calories: 560, Protein: 36g, Carbohydrate: 92g, Fat: 9g

**Snack/Dessert** _____

1 oz. dry roasted peanuts

Calories: 160, Protein: 5g, Carbohydrate: 7g, Fat: 13g

## WEEK SIX, DAY FIVE

**Breakfast** _____ or _____ **Quick Fix Breakfast**

2 eggs, hard-boiled or ½ c. egg substitute, scrambled

1 slice whole-grain toast with low-sugar jelly

½ c. low-fat yogurt

Calories: 322, Protein: 21g, Carbohydrate: 44g, Fat: 11g

Denny's® Fit Fair™ Veggie Omelette with English Muffin (dry)

Calories: 330, Protein: 25g, Carbohydrate: 37g, Fat: 8g

**Snack** _____ or _____ **Quick Fix Snack**

1 oz. low-fat mozzarella cheese

2 rice cakes

1 c. strawberries

Calories: 206, Protein: 9g, Carbohydrate: 27g, Fat: 5g

McDonald's® Yogurt Parfait

Calories: 160, Protein: 4g, Carbohydrate: 31g, Fat: 2g

**Lunch** _____ or _____ **Quick Fix Lunch**

2 oz. turkey breast and 1 oz. low-fat cheese in small whole-wheat pita

2 c. romaine lettuce with ½ c. orange slices, 2 T. raisins, and 1 T. low-fat salad dressing

Calories: 322, Protein: 25g, Carbohydrate: 24g, Fat: 14g

Ruby Tuesday® Skinny Chicken Salad

Calories: 283, Protein: 38g, Carbohydrate: 10g, Fat: 10g

**Snack** _____

1 packet Quaker® Instant Oatmeal, Lower Sugar Apples & Cinnamon

1 c. light yogurt

Calories: 190, Protein: 10g, Carbohydrate: 39g, Fat: 1g

**Dinner** _____ or _____ **Quick Fix Dinner**

6 oz. baked cod with lemon herb seasoning

1 c. grilled onions and peppers

1 c. sautéed green beans in 1 T. light margarine

1 small baked sweet potato with 1 T. light margarine

Calories: 584, Protein: 50g, Carbohydrate: 49g, Fat: 20g

*Frozen*

Stouffer's® Grilled Herb Chicken

1 c. baby carrots with 2 T. low-fat dressing

Calories: 351, Protein: 21g, Carbohydrate: 42g, Fat: 11g

or

*Restaurant*

Blimpie® Grille Max with cheese

Calories: 510, Protein: 25g, Carbohydrate: 71g, Fat: 11g

**Snack/Dessert** _____

½ c. low-fat cottage cheese

½ c. sliced apricots

Calories: 161, Protein: 16g, Carbohydrate: 21g, Fat: 2g

## WEEK SIX, DAY SIX

**Breakfast** _____ or _____ **Quick Fix Breakfast**

Power shake: Mix 1 scoop whey protein
powder, 1 c. blueberries, ½ c. low-fat
berry yogurt, and ½ c. nonfat milk

Calories: 345, Protein: 35g, Carbohydrate: 44g, Fat: 1g

Yoplait® Nouriche Drink (11 oz.)

Calories: 260, Protein: 10g, Carbohydrate: 55g, Fat: 0g

**Snack** _____ or _____ **Quick Fix Snack**

½ c. low-fat cottage cheese
1 c. sliced peaches

Calories: 201, Protein: 14g, Carbohydrate: 32g, Fat: 2g

1 apple
10 almonds

Calories: 129, Protein: 4g, Carbohydrate: 17g, Fat: 6g

**Lunch** _____ or _____ **Quick Fix Lunch**

Salad of: 3 oz. grilled chicken breast, 1 c.
fresh baby spinach, and ½ c. sliced
mushrooms with 2 T. low-fat sweet and
sour dressing
6 whole-wheat crackers

Calories: 312, Protein: 23g, Carbohydrate: 24g, Fat: 14g

Healthy Choice® Meatloaf

Calories: 300, Protein: 15g, Carbohydrate: 40g, Fat: 8g

**Snack** _____

Low-fat whole-grain nutrition bar

Calories: 140, Protein: 5g, Carbohydrate: 23g, Fat: 2g

**Dinner** _____ or _____ **Quick Fix Dinner**

6 oz. baked Italian marinated chicken
(marinate in low-fat Italian dressing for
30–60 min.)
1½ c. cooked green beans with ½ T. light
margarine and 1 T. slivered almonds
1 c. whole-wheat pasta with ½ T. light
margarine

Calories: 590, Protein: 57g, Carbohydrate: 63g, Fat: 16g

*Frozen*

Stouffer's® Beef Pot Roast
½ c. sliced peaches
6 oz. light yogurt

Calories: 360, Protein: 23g, Carbohydrate: 49g, Fat: 8g

or

*Restaurant*

Boston Market® Roasted Sirloin (5 oz.)
4.7 oz. green beans
3.9 oz. mashed potatoes (equals ½ serving),
no gravy

Calories: 495, Protein: 44g, Carbohydrate: 27g, Fat: 25g

**Snack/Dessert** _____

1 oz. low-fat cheese
1 c. fresh blueberries

Calories: 148, Protein: 8g, Carbohydrate: 17g, Fat: 5g

## WEEK SIX, DAY SEVEN

**Breakfast** _____ or _____ **Quick Fix Breakfast**

2 slices whole-wheat toast with 2 slices
melted low-fat mozzarella cheese
4 to 6 slices tomato

Calories: 300, Protein: 18g, Carbohydrate: 40g, Fat: 8g

Myoplex® Lite Ready-to-Drink Shake or
similar product
1 large peach

Calories: 251, Protein: 26g, Carbohydrate: 35g, Fat: 3g

**Snack** _____ or _____ **Quick Fix Snack**

1 egg, hard-boiled
6 low-sodium saltine crackers
1 medium pear

Calories: 220, Protein: 9g, Carbohydrate: 30g, Fat: 7g

1½ oz. tropical trail mix

Calories: 171, Protein: 3g, Carbohydrate: 28g, Fat: 7g

**Lunch** _____ or _____ **Quick Fix Lunch**

2 oz. lean ham and 1 oz. low-fat cheese
with 2 T. low-fat dressing
¼ c. dried cranberries

Calories: 347, Protein: 33g, Carbohydrate: 38g, Fat: 7g

Lean Cuisine® Chicken in Peanut Sauce

Calories: 280, Protein: 22g, Carbohydrate: 30g, Fat: 8g

**Snack** _____

1 oz. roasted almonds

Calories: 150, Protein: 8g, Carbohydrate: 4g, Fat: 12g

**Dinner** _____ or _____ **Quick Fix Dinner**

6 oz. grilled pork tenderloin
2 c. steamed cauliflower, snap peas, and
broccoli with 1 T. light margarine
⅔ c. cooked brown rice

Calories: 553, Protein: 58g, Carbohydrate: 43g, Fat: 14g

*Frozen*
Stouffer's® Skillets Steak Teriyaki
1 medium apple
1 oz. low-fat cheese

Calories: 430, Protein: 25g, Carbohydrate: 60g, Fat: 10g

or

*Restaurant*
Applebee's® Teriyaki Steak 'n Shrimp Skewers

Calories: 450, Protein: 47g, Carbohydrate: 48g, Fat: 8g

**Snack/Dessert** _____

½ c. fat-free sorbet
1 T. low-fat granola

Calories: 160, Protein: 1g, Carbohydrate: 37g, Fat: 1g

# CHAPTER 8

# Smart Exercise

*I have a couple of five-pound weights in my office, and when I feel myself tensing up, sometimes I'll shut the door and do some bicep curls, just to get the blood flowing and circulating.*

—SUSAN SOLOVIC, CEO AND CHAIRMAN OF SBTV.COM

## ONE-MINUTE SUMMARY

- Lifting weights helps you look and feel better and, when done correctly, makes your body better at doing everyday activities and staying injury free.
- Muscles consist of two types of fiber—slow twitch (or Type I) for endurance and fast twitch (or Type II) for power.
- Resistance exercise actually damages these muscle fibers, but they repair themselves by laying down tiny protein filaments, which grow stronger and bigger. Increased musculature then boosts your metabolism.
- An exercise program should strengthen your body's power center—the core, which is the muscles of the abdomen, spine, hips, and pelvis.

I f you've already launched the Quick-Start Action Plan from Chapter 2, put some thought into your health and fitness vision from Chapter 5, and begun the Entrepreneur Diet in Chapter 7, you've made bigger strides than most people ever will.

Now we'll get down to the nuts and bolts of an effective exercise program. Because your time is at a premium, this routine can be done in the comfort of your home or even in your office, in as few as two days a week. The only equipment required is a set of dumbbells. These exercises—based on cutting-edge principles from the National Academy of Sports Medicine (NASM)—build muscle as well as improve your balance and strengthen your "core," the all-important midsection of the body that often gets ignored in other exercise routines.

The program comes in a progression of two phases—Level 1 and Level 2, which we'll look at later in this chapter. As a result, you develop your fitness in a way that gets results while minimizing the risk of overdoing things.

## WEIGHT LIFTING DEMYSTIFIED

In recent years, weight lifting has evolved to become something more than a way to get big biceps. Nowadays, while building a better body certainly still is a goal, the focus also includes improving the function of muscles in everyday movements and staying injury free. That's a good thing given that more of us are working in offices, sitting for hours every day, and moving less and less. This adds up to muscular imbalances, tightness, and injuries when we do move—in fact, low-back pain afflicts about 80 percent of the adult population.

And so as the benefits of exercising the body's muscles gain greater awareness, resistance training is no longer reserved for elite athletes and the burly guys

## TERMINOLOGY TAKE

Instead of talking about "weight lifting," exercise scientists often refer to "resistance training" or "resistance exercise"—because the resistance doesn't have to be provided by a dumbbell or a weight; it can be supplied by your body, as with a push-up or a squat (sometimes called a deep knee bend).

banging barbells around. Increasingly, resistance training is seen as a way for people of all ages, shapes, and sizes to look and feel better, and to improve everyday functioning.

### *Muscle Basics*

Your body contains more than 430 skeletal muscles, each made up of a bundle of individual muscle fibers. These fibers can be broken down into two basic types: slow twitch (or Type I) and fast twitch (or Type II). Slow-twitch fibers, as the name implies, contract gradually. Although smaller in size and unable to generate as much force as fast-twitch fibers, slow-twitch fibers have high endurance. These fibers are important for stabilizing your body and maintaining your posture—when you're sitting upright, for example.

Fast-twitch fibers contract quickly, are larger, and can produce greater force than the slow-twitch variety, but they're not as efficient at using oxygen and tire more quickly. When you've sprinted from a standstill to get across a street without getting hit by traffic, you can thank your fast-twitch fibers for getting you to the other side without being flattened.

All muscles have a mix of slow- and fast-twitch fibers—the proportions depend on which muscle you're considering, as explained in NASM's *Optimum Performance Training for the Health and Fitness Professional: Course Manual, 2nd edition*, 2004. Your shin muscle, for example, is made up of about 73 percent slow twitch, while your calf muscle is made up of about 50 percent slow twitch.

---

**TIME SAVER TIP**

If you belong to a health club, keep a set of workout clothes and shoes in your car so you're always ready for the gym. Or pay for a locker—and a laundry service, if available—so you have clean workout clothes there all the time, advises Claire Gruppo, founder and CEO of New York-based investment banking firm Gruppo, Levey & Co. "No excuses!" she says.

---

### Muscling Up

When you exercise your muscles, they adapt by getting bigger and stronger (although muscle size gains tend to vary by individual and, as mentioned in Chapter 3, by gender). It's your body's way of meeting the challenge you're giving it.

How does this happen? Ironically, exercising a muscle actually damages muscle fibers—but they don't stay damaged. They undergo a repair and remodeling process that is aided by a release of hormones and adds tiny protein filaments to increase the overall size of the muscle.

Those bigger muscles don't just give a new look to your body, they speed up your metabolism. Muscle is more metabolically active than fat—so when you build muscle, you increase your "internal furnace" and burn more calories throughout the day, even when you're not exercising.

### Core and Balance

Exercising your muscles in the right way also can strengthen your body's "core," which is the center part of your body. In addition to your abdominal muscles, the

---

## RESISTANCE TRAINING AND THE HEART

Walking and running usually are cited as good ways to boost your cardiovascular health. But resistance training also may play a role in enhancing the cardiovascular system. Two small studies from the 1980s on people with high blood pressure showed decreases in resting blood pressure following a weight training program. And in a study of adults age 60 to 83 published in 2002 in *Archives of Internal Medicine*, a six-month resistance training program improved their body's ability to use oxygen by at least 20 percent. The participants also increased by about 25 percent the time they could walk on a treadmill before tiring.

A caveat: Lifting very heavy weight (the equivalent of your body weight when bench pressing, for example) can put high stress on the heart. Those with a family history of aneurysms and people older than age 40 should take greater care when lifting heavy weights.

---

core encompasses the spine, hips, and pelvic muscles. It includes deeper-level muscles (consisting mostly of slow-twitch fibers) that help to stabilize your body and form a foundation for your movement. "In layman's terms, the core is everything but your arms and legs," says Tyler Wallace, a performance-enhancement specialist and corrective-exercise specialist at NASM.

> *The stronger my core is, the less likely I am to have any kind of back trouble. And everything else just seems to function better.*
>
> —TERRI ALPERT, FOUNDER AND CEO OF UNO ALLA VOLTA LLC

A weak core can lead to injury, including lower-back problems. And without a strong core, the strength of your arms and legs is diminished. Think about a golf swing. The power of the leg drive has to travel through the trunk of the body to reach the shoulders and arms swinging the club. If the core is weak, this transfer of energy runs into a roadblock.

And yet, the deeper core muscles are often completely ignored in exercise programs. As explained in NASM's *Course Manual*, not training these muscles is like "building a house without a foundation."

The exercises described in this chapter include movements that target core muscles by challenging your ability to stabilize and balance—maneuvering on one foot, for example. And these balance exercises have a bonus feature; they burn extra calories. Why? Because your body is exercising in an unstable environment, it's forced to use more muscles and so it expends more calories.

## THE RESISTANCE PROGRAM

This innovative NASM-based workout requires only a pair of dumbbells, and you'll get a full-body workout in a minimal amount of time. Make sure you follow these guidelines:

- The program is divided into two six-week phases—Level 1 and Level 2. If you're new to exercise or coming back from time off, begin with Level 1. If you're an experienced exerciser, start with Level 2. At first, aim for two exercise sessions a week, with at least one day off between sessions. When you begin Level 2, consider adding a third day—although it's not necessary.

## CAN YOU HEAR ME NOW?

Listening to music in your iPod while you lift weights can be motivating, but whether it's good for your ears is another matter. Listening for extended periods at high volumes can lead to gradual hearing loss—in fact, you may not realize the damage until your hearing is too far gone. Noise that registers more than 85 decibels (dB) can result in a permanent loss of hearing, according to the American Speech-Hearing-Language Association (ASHA). Portable listening devices can hit up to 120 dB, ASHA warns—this is comparable to snowmobile noise and can lead to damaged hearing after just 7½ minutes of listening.

In addition to keeping down the volume and limiting your listening time, ASHA recommends that you consider trading the earbuds, which rest inside the ear, for noise-canceling headphones that surround the ear. They may be a little more awkward to work out with, but by reducing background noise, you won't be as tempted to crank up the volume and jeopardize your hearing.

- In Chapter 4, you identified muscle imbalances you may have with the NASM Overhead Squat Assessment. Take a minute to look at your self-assessment results on pages 61–62. Later in this chapter is a description of the exercises and a note of which muscle imbalance checkpoints a particular exercise will help address. You should still perform all of the exercises—this information is provided so that you are more aware of how the exercises benefit you. After four or six weeks, you should see marked improvement in the Overhead Squat Assessment.
- You can pick up dumbbells at a local sporting goods store or order them online. A pair of 15-pound dumbbells runs about $20. Adjustable dumbbells—such as PowerBlocks®, ProBell® adjustable dumbbell system, and Bowflex® SelectTech™ dumbbells—allow you to change the weight on a single set of dumbbells and start at about $120 (visit www.performbetter.com and www.nautilus.com). AquaBells® are collapsible travel dumbbells that fit neatly into your luggage—you fill them up with water at your destination to

create up to 16 pounds of weight per dumbbell ($60 for a pair; visit www .aquabells.com).

- While you perform each exercise, do the "drawing in" maneuver you learned about in Chapter 2—a small inward movement of pulling the belly button toward the spine. "This will activate the transverse abdominis and other core muscles," Wallace explains. "In essence, you're tightening the midsection. This serves to strengthen the core and also enhances strength throughout the rest of the body as you perform the exercise."

- Rest for about a minute between exercises. Initially, you may not want to use any weight at all, just to get a feel for the movements. As you progress, where dumbbells are required, use a weight that you can lift for 12 to 15 repetitions, but no more, before tiring (recall that a "repetition" or "rep" is one complete movement of a given exercise, and a "set" is a given number repetitions done in sequence). No matter what, don't use a weight that causes your form to break down.

- For exercises done while standing on two feet, stand with your feet about shoulder-width apart, toes pointed straight ahead, and keep a very slight flex in your knees.

- At the end of the three-month program, take one week off—your body will benefit from the rest and will come back even stronger when you return to the gym. You can return to Level 2 or start again with Level 1.

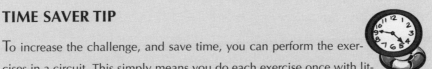

**TIME SAVER TIP**

To increase the challenge, and save time, you can perform the exercises in a circuit. This simply means you do each exercise once with little or no rest in between, then return to the first exercise to perform the entire circuit again. Big warning here, though: don't try this until you have several months of exercising under your belt because it's strenuous.

---

## BACK IN THE GAME

Business owner Robert Smith had been an athlete in college, but after graduation had gotten away from fitness. He says being out of shape can manifest itself in subtle ways. "It was affecting my performance at work because I was fatigued all the time," he explains. "I didn't have the energy to keep going. Even when sitting at the computer, you're still active—getting files, grasping a book—but I just got tired." When Smith hit his lifetime high weight, he decided to do something about it, limiting his calorie intake and running twice a day. Soon, he had slimmed down. "I look and feel better than I did when I was 21," he says. He draws an analogy between his tough workout mentality and his business life. "It all goes hand in hand," he says. "I bring my killer-instinct attitude that I have in the gym to the office."

---

### *Level 1*

The first six weeks of the program are designed to enhance the stability of your joints, improve your posture, and build muscle. You do core and balance exercises, as well as resistance exercises for each of the major body parts—chest, back, shoulders, arms, and legs. For the first one or two weeks, perform just one set per exercise. As you progress, you can add a second set.

### *Level 2*

In Level 2, you'll build on your progress in Level 1 with exercises that target functional strength and provide even greater balance challenges (some of the exercises require that you lift one foot off the ground). You could start here if you're already an experienced exerciser. Aim for two or three sets per exercise.

### THE EXERCISES

All photos are courtesy of Karen Thomas of Entrepreneur Press and photographer Julia Cappelli.

## *Core and Balance*

### TWO-LEG FLOOR BRIDGE (LEVEL 1)

*Targets imbalances around the feet, knees, and low back*

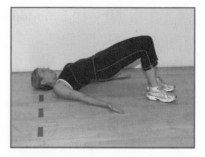

FIGURE 8.1: **Two-Leg Floor Bridge**

Lie on your back with your knees bent and feet flat on the floor, shoulder-width apart. Angle your arms out to the side, with palms up. Now press through your heels and lift your hips off the floor so your knees, hips, and shoulders form a straight line (see Figure 8.1). Hold for about 5 seconds and slowly lower to the starting position, and repeat.

*To make more difficult:* Perform with one foot slightly off the floor.

### SINGLE-LEG BALANCE (LEVEL 1)

*Targets imbalances around the feet, knees, and low back*

Standing with your hands on your hips (see Figure 8.2A), lift your left foot a few inches off the ground, slightly flexing your knee and flexing your foot toward your shin (see Figure 8.2B). Hold for 5 to 10 seconds and slowly lower to the starting position. Repeat with right leg.

FIGURE 8.2: **Single-Leg Balance**

A. Start

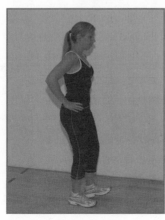

B. Movement

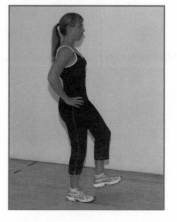

### QUADRUPED LIMB RAISE (LEVEL 2)

*Targets imbalances around the feet, knees, low back, and shoulders*

FIGURE 8.3: **Quadruped Limb Raise**

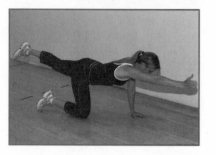

Begin on your hands and knees, with your back in its natural curve. Pull your abs in and tuck your chin. Gently raise both your right arm (thumb pointed up) and your left leg (toes aimed away from your body). Keep both limbs straight and about even with your torso (see Figure 8.3). Think of "reaching long." Hold for a second or two, then slowly return to the starting position. Repeat with opposite limbs. This is one rep.

*To make easier:* Raise one limb at a time.

### CRUNCH (LEVEL 2)

*Targets imbalances around the low back*

Lie on your back with your knees bent and feet flat on the ground. Position your arms over your chest (see Figure 8.4A), pull in your abs and slowly curl your torso upward. Think of moving your belly button toward your hips (see Figure 8.4B). Slowly return to the starting position and repeat.

FIGURE 8.4: **Crunch**

A. Start

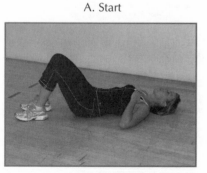

B. Movement

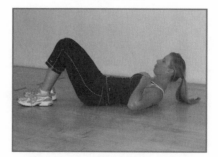

### *Resistance*

PUSH-UP, STANDARD OR MODIFIED (LEVEL 1)

*Targets imbalances around the shoulders*

Begin in the standard push-up position, with hands a little wider than your shoulders (see Figure 8.5A). Bend your elbows to slowly lower toward the ground, maintaining a flat back. Lower until your upper arms are about parallel to the ground (see Figure 8.5B), then push back to the start and repeat. Keep your head in a natural position—not flexing forward or extending up.

*To modify and make easier:* Perform with your knees on the ground, or your hands up on a bench or desk and feet touching the floor.

UNEVEN PUSH-UP (LEVEL 2)

*Targets imbalances around the shoulders*

Perform a push-up with one hand placed on a large book or a softball. Or if you have a medicine ball, place one hand on the medicine ball (alternate the uneven hand from set-to-set).

STANDING DUMBBELL ROW (LEVEL 1)

*Targets imbalances around the shoulders*

Grasp a dumbbell in each hand. Bend from the waist so that your upper torso maintains a 45-degree angle to the floor, with weights hanging down toward the knees (see Figure 8.6A). Pull the dumbbells straight up to your sides until your upper arms are about parallel with the ground, squeezing your shoulder blades together

FIGURE 8.5: **Push-Up**

A. Start

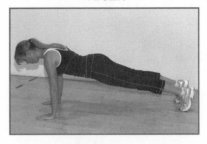

B. Movement

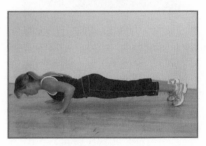

FIGURE 8.6: **Standing Dumbbell Row**

A. Start

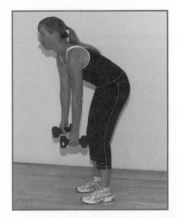

FIGURE 8.6: **Standing Dumbbell Row**

B. Movement

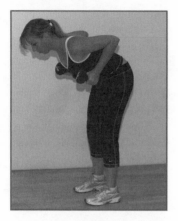

and keeping the elbows in toward your body (see Figure 8.6B). Slowly return to the start and repeat.

*To make easier:* Decrease the bend at your waist.

SINGLE-LEG DUMBBELL ROW (LEVEL 2)
*Targets imbalances around the feet, knees, low back, and shoulders*
Perform a standing dumbbell row on one leg (on left leg for one set, on right leg for the next).

STANDING DUMBBELL MILITARY PRESS (LEVEL 1)
*Targets imbalances around the shoulders*
Grasp a dumbbell in each hand and stand straight. Flex your elbows and hold the dumbbells with forearms perpendicular to the ground, palms facing to the front (see Figure 8.7A). Straighten your arms overhead, with palms still facing out (see Figure 8.7B). Slowly return to the start and repeat.

SINGLE-LEG DUMBBELL MILITARY PRESS (LEVEL 2)
*Targets imbalances around the shoulders*
Perform the dumbbell military press on one leg (on left leg for one set, on right leg for the next).

FIGURE 8.7: **Standing Dumbbell Military Press**

A. Start

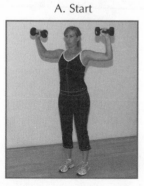

B. Movement

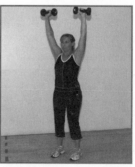

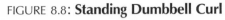

STANDING DUMBBELL CURL (LEVEL 1)

*Targets the upper arms (but not specific imbalances identified in Chapter 4)*

Grasp a dumbbell in each hand and stand straight. Your arms should be hanging down at your sides, with palms facing to the front (see Figure 8.8A). Flex your elbows to curl the dumbbells up to the front of your shoulders, with palms facing your body. Keep your elbows close to your sides throughout the movement (see Figure 8.8B). Slowly return to the starting position and repeat.

FIGURE 8.8: **Standing Dumbbell Curl**

A. Start

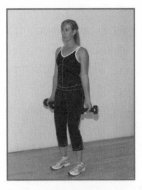

B. Movement

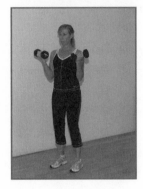

SINGLE-LEG DUMBBELL CURL (LEVEL 2)

*Targets imbalances around the feet, knees, and low back*

Perform a standing dumbbell curl on one leg—on left leg for one set, on right leg for the next (see Figure 8.9A and B).

FIGURE 8.9: **Single-Leg Dumbbell Curl**

A. Start

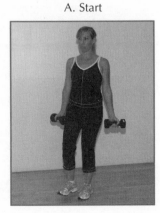

B. Movement

FIGURE 8.10: **Step-Up to Balance**

A. Start

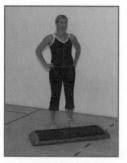

B. Movement

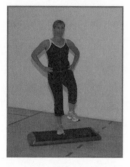

STEP-UP TO BALANCE (LEVEL 1)
*Targets imbalances around the feet, knees, and low back*

Face a step or a box between 6 and 18 inches high. Stand tall, pull in your abs, and tighten your glutes (see Figure 8.10A). Step up onto the step with your right foot. Lift your left leg, with the left knee and hip flexed to about 90 degrees (see Figure 8.10B). You should be balancing on just your right foot on the box. Hold for a second, then return your left foot to the floor, followed by your right foot (this is one repetition). Repeat, this time with your right foot raised in the air.

SQUAT, CURL, AND PRESS (LEVEL 2)
*Targets imbalances around the feet, knees, low back, and shoulders*

Stand straight and grasp a dumbbell in each hand, holding them at your sides. Squat down slowly, as if you were taking a seat in a chair, until your knees are flexed to about 90 degrees or until your spine starts

FIGURE 8.11: **Squat, Curl, and Press**

A. Squat Movement

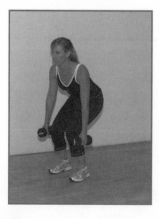

B. Curl Movement

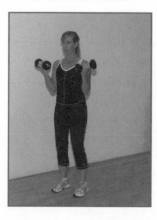

C. Overhead Press Movement

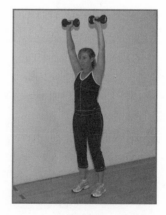

to lose its natural curve (see Figure 8.11A). Press through your heels to return to the starting position. Next, perform a dumbbell curl (see Figure 8.11B). Then press the dumbbells above your head until your arms are straight, rotating the weights so that your palms face out (see Figure 8.11C). Slowly return to the starting position (dumbbells at sides), then repeat.

*To make easier:* Don't use weights

---

### *Action* Items

➤ If you don't have any weights, this week purchase a pair of dumbbells at a sporting goods store or online (visit www.performbetter.com or www.nautilus.com).

➤ Determine the best days and times of the week to work out, and schedule two sessions for this week as you would business meetings. Leave at least a day between workouts. Do the same the following week (try to make the days and times consistent week to week).

➤ If you like, make the first few workout days a trial run through the exercises, without weights, to get a feel for the movements.

---

## WORKOUT BOX

### Level 1 (Weeks 1–6; perform the workout two times a week)

| Exercise | Repetitions | Sets |
|---|---|---|
| **Core and Balance** | | |
| Two-leg floor bridge | 12 | 1–2 |
| Single-leg balance | 6–10 per leg | 1–2 |
| **Resistance** | | |
| Push-up, standard or modified | 12–15 | 1–2 |
| Standing dumbbell row | 12–15 | 1–2 |
| Standing dumbbell military press | 12–15 | 1–2 |
| Standing dumbbell curl | 12–15 | 1–2 |
| Step-up to balance | 12–15 | 1–2 |

### Level 2 (Weeks 7–12; perform the workout two or three times a week)

| Exercise | Repetitions | Sets |
|---|---|---|
| **Core and Balance** | | |
| Quadruped limb raise | 6–10 | 2–3 |
| Crunch | 15–20 | 2–3 |
| **Resistance** | | |
| Squat, curl, and press | 12–15 | 2–3 |
| Uneven push-up | 12–15 | 2–3 |
| Single-leg dumbbell row | 12–15 | 2–3 |
| Single-leg dumbbell military press | 12–15 | 2–3 |
| Single-leg dumbbell curl | 12–15 | 2–3 |

# CHAPTER 9

# Cardio Matters

*I schedule exercise in my day to give myself a mental break, whether it's a jog outside, a treadmill run, or a swim . . . These sessions are critical to my sanity in terms of letting off steam.*

—Margaret Moore, founder and CEO of Wellcoaches Corporation

## ONE-MINUTE SUMMARY

🕐 When you build on the foundation of the ten-minute energy walk, in three months you'll boost your endurance and run for 30 minutes at a time.

🕐 Aerobic exercise helps control weight and causes healthy changes in your body—for example, your heart pumps more blood with each beat, the diameter of your blood vessels increases, and blood pressure may drop.

🕐 Mentally, doing aerobic exercise boosts your mood and energy.

🕐 A pair of running shoes cushions the impact of your foot striking the ground, and a sports watch offers an easy way to time your sessions.

> ⏱ Your aerobic plan involves three sessions each week, progressing from easy to medium to hard so that your body can grow ever stronger but also have time to recover.

The human body is made to move. On the outside, the synergy of the arms, legs, and torso propels you forward, while support systems on the inside supply the energy to make it possible. Like the employees of a company that's running smoothly, the parts of your body get better at what they do by working together over time, improving the ways in which they communicate and interact with each other. And like a company whose profits rise as employees gain experience, the health of your body improves as your heart and lungs are put to work.

If you've done the ten-minute energy walks as part of the Quick-Start Action Plan from Chapter 2, you're already on your way to taking the next step in aerobic fitness. This chapter gives you a fast overview of how your aerobic systems work and then launches you on an easy-to-implement cardio program. You'll steadily increase your endurance so that by the end of three months you're able to run for 30 minutes at a time. And if running isn't your thing, you'll discover some other effective options.

## TEAM CARDIO

Aerobic exercise is a highly effective way to manage your weight—depending on your size and pace, walking can burn about 400 calories per hour, while running can burn twice that. What, exactly, is aerobic exercise? It's activity done for an extended period of time at an increased heart rate, and typically involves repeatedly and rhythmically moving large muscles in your legs and arms. Aerobic means "with oxygen," in that the body uses oxygen to generate energy. Sometimes aerobic exercise is referred to as "cardiovascular exercise" or simply "cardio."

Although muscles and bones do the heavy lifting when you move, it's the heart, veins, arteries, and lungs that provide the engine to drive your motion. As you breathe in, air is warmed and moistened, moving down the trachea and eventually to hundreds of millions of microscopic structures in the lungs. From there, oxygen moves into the bloodstream, traveling to the heart to be pumped out to the body's tissues.

At the same time, the bloodstream transports carbon dioxide—a waste by-product of cell metabolism—in the reverse direction. Carbon dioxide moves from the cells to the heart, eventually making it to the lungs and back outside through exhalation. In short, the heart, blood, and lungs provide a 24/7 conveyer belt of oxygen and carbon dioxide so the body's trillions (yes, *trillions*) of cells can perform their critical functions, including muscle contraction.

And through regular aerobic exercise, this physiological machinery becomes more efficient at its job.

## GROWING STRONGER

As you become more aerobically fit, for example, your heart gets better at pumping blood and delivering oxygen throughout your body. In fact, aerobic exercise can boost the amount of blood your heart pumps with each beat, meaning your heart doesn't have to work as hard to keep blood circulating. As mentioned in Chapter 4, while the average person's ticker beats between 60 to 80 times per minute at rest, trained athletes can have heart rates of 40 beats per minute.

### A NATURAL PAIN KILLER

Intuitively, you might think that exercise is rough on the joints—especially as you get older. But research indicates that the opposite is true. Vigorous exercise may actually decrease the pains that come with aging, according to a 2005 study published in *Arthritis Research & Therapy*. For a period of 14 years, researchers kept tabs on 492 members of a runners association and 374 nonmembers. All the subjects participating in the study were at least 50 years old. The conclusion: although fractures happened with slightly more frequency among runners, they also reported experiencing about 25 percent less pain than the nonrunners.

To put these numbers in a different perspective, think about this: if you lower your heart rate by 10 beats per minute, you'll save more than 5 million heartbeats in the next year. In the next 10 years, that's more than 50 million heartbeats.

Aerobic exercise causes even more beneficial changes.

- Your body generates more capillaries—tiny blood vessels that help transfer oxygen and carbon dioxide.
- The diameter of blood vessels increases, allowing for an easier flow of blood.
- The volume of blood plasma in your body rises by about 20 percent.
- Your muscles become better at extracting oxygen from the bloodstream to produce energy.

With all this happening, it's not unusual to have blood pressure decrease with aerobic exercise—and this may happen very quickly. In a study out of Ireland published in 2006, researchers put 17 young, healthy men on a four-week training program that involved stationary cycling for 30 minutes three or four times a week. After just one week of training, their blood pressure at rest had fallen significantly—from an average of 121/66 mmHg to 110/57 mmHg (mmHg stands for millimeters of mercury).

When these physiological changes take place, you can find a new appreciation for what your body can achieve. In *The Elements of Effort: Reflections on the Art and Science of Running* (Pocket Books, 1997), writer and runner John Jerome describes his own revelation: "The training effect itself—the body's natural improvement in response to stress—is the most delicious small piece of physiology I know. I wouldn't have learned about it if it weren't for running."

## INSTANT BOOSTER

Given this interaction between the mind and the exercising body, it makes sense that an enhanced feeling of energy is usually the result of a walk, run, bike ride, or swim—both during your session and for some time afterward. In fact, a study from the late 1970s found that running can be as effective as psychotherapy in helping with depression. And the early mental benefits of aerobic exercise can be long-lasting. In a study of depressed adults published in 1999 in the journal *Preventive Medicine*, researchers found that the improved moods the participants enjoyed

## THE FIT BRAIN

Getting out for a walk may not just improve your mood; it also may help ward off Alzheimer's disease. A 2004 study of more than 16,000 women age 70 to 81 published in the *Journal of the American Medical Association* found that those who walked 90 minutes a week did better on mental function tests than less active women. A second 2004 study, also published in *JAMA*, looked at more than 2,000 men age 71 to 93. Those who took daily walks of more than two miles had almost half the risk of developing dementia compared with men who put on their walking shoes for under a quarter-mile per day.

after a 12-week stationary bike exercise program were still present 12 months later (the researchers assumed the subjects kept up their training).

It's not entirely clear where this mental boost comes from. One explanation is an increased release of endorphins after exercise. Endorphins are linked to a positive mood and an improved sense of well-being. Another reason may be that exercise increases certain neurotransmitters in the brain (such as serotonin and dopamine) that show low levels during depression. Still other reasons could be that exercise simply distracts a person from negative thoughts or instills a feeling of self-efficacy—the confidence to accomplish a task.

Aerobic exercise has another potential mood-lifting benefit—getting outdoors during winter exposes you to sunlight, which may help relieve the effects of seasonal affective disorder or SAD. This condition can cause depression during the winter months, when the shorter and darker days stimulate the body to produce more melatonin, a hormone implicated in causing depressive symptoms. (For more information on SAD, visit the National Mental Health Association at www.nmha.org.)

## THE CARDIO PROGRAM

With the benefits of cardiovascular exercise firmly in mind, it's time to get started. This is a three-month, step-by-step plan (set out at the end of the chapter) to take you from short walks to 30 minutes of continuous running. Your goal for the first week is ten minutes of walking for three days. That's it. If you've completed the energy-walk portion in the Quick-Start Action Plan, you've already begun!

## AN EDUCATION IN RUNNING

Business owner Stephen Gatlin began a regular running program several years ago, and now his jogs have become a welcome habit. "I look forward to it," he says. "If I skip a workout, it's not so much guilt that I feel, but I regret missing out on that time that I've set aside for myself."

Running helps him solve work issues and improve his focus, he says, and for someone with a driven type-A personality, running also creates a nice calming effect. "I'm sure all my employees really appreciate my running," he laughs. "It keeps you from being crazed." The native Texan runs every other day, covering about 20 miles a week, and also does three or four half-marathon events during the winter months.

Gatlin's company, Gatlin Education Services, started providing education on the internet in 1994, and today the Fort Worth, Texas-based company is the largest provider of online, instructor-supported training to colleges and universities.

Gatlin has gone through periods of being overweight, but now weighs 190 pounds on a 6-foot-three-inch frame. Although he watches his diet, he's not fanatical about it, he says. He figures his running allows him some dietary splurges now and then. "I look at running as an antidote for indulgence—maybe having that good cheeseburger, instead of just trying to follow a perfect diet," he says. (Research backs him up—data collected on more than 7,000 men in the 1990s, as part of the National Runners' Health Study, indicated that the more a person runs, the less effect their diet choices have on body fat.)

His advice for starting a fitness program? "You have to make exercise a priority," he says. Plan exercise the night before—what your workout will be and where—and stick to your guns. "You can't change your mind, otherwise, certainly in the early stages, you'll have no chance."

## THE TREADMILL TEST

A long-term study by researchers at Northwestern University in Illinois, looking at thousands of young adults, found that people who did poorly on a treadmill test were twice as likely than their fitter peers to get high blood pressure or diabetes 15 years later. But there's good news—you can make a comeback. Some of the study participants performed a second treadmill test seven years after the first. Those who showed improved fitness during those seven years decreased their risk of diabetes by 40 percent.

By starting slowly, you prepare your body to handle more later. "The first thing you have to do is build a base, just like you do with weight training," explains Paul Robbins, who consults with the National Academy of Sports Medicine on its cardiovascular-exercise curriculum and trains elite athletes at Athletes' Performance in Tempe, Arizona. Robbins also provides expert consulting for employee wellness programs at Adidas and TJX (the parent company of T.J. Maxx and Marshalls stores). Beginning in the third week, start to include short jogs during your walks, and as the weeks go on, gradually intersperse more running with your walking—until eventually you're just running.

Generally, within each week you progress from easier to harder workouts (see pages 177–178). You'll notice that Mondays typically involve the shortest workouts, while Fridays feature the longest. By rotating from lower-demand to higher-demand sessions, Robbins says, you progressively challenge your body but also allow it time to recover—and grow ever stronger. "By staying in the rotation of low-, medium-, and high-demand workouts," he adds, "you won't get burned out."

If you already have a regular walking program and want to start running, begin with the third month of the program. Or if you'd like to begin a walking program but don't desire to run, you can still use the plan—simply substitute more vigorous walking in place of the running portions of each session. The extra effort will have you burning more calories.

Now, let's look at some tips to keep in mind as you get started.

## BORN TO RUN?

A study published in *Nature* in 2004 concluded that our prehistoric ancestors' need to run long distances, maybe for hunting and scavenging, shaped our very anatomy. For example, humans have large surface areas in the hip, knee, and ankle joints, making for better shock absorption while running because the impact forces are spread out.

### If the Shoe Fits

If you don't have running shoes, buy a pair—the cushioning helps protect your joints. Find a store that specializes in running and try out several pairs by jogging around the store. You'll likely wear a larger size than you do with your regular shoes—aim for about a thumb's-width of space between the front of the shoe and your longest toe.

### Figure Out Logistics

You can walk and run outside or indoors on a treadmill. If you head outside, pick a flat, out-and-back course so it's easier to stick close to the prescribed times. (If you are curious about how far you are going measure your route online at www .usatf.org/routes/map. )Invest in a sports watch with a built-in stopwatch to make timing your sessions straightforward—a Timex® Ironman®-style watch is a good choice and retails for about $50 (visit www.timex.com).

### Warm Up and Cool Down

It's important to start any running or walking session with easy walking or jogging for a few minutes. This gets blood to your muscles and allows them to warm up. Going too fast right off the bat can lead to injury because you're stressing cold muscles. Toward the end of your session, spend a couple of minutes doing slower walking/jogging.

### *Expect to Feel Sluggish*

When your body goes from a resting state—say sitting at your desk—to an active state, it takes a while to adjust to that "shock to the system." So expect the first minutes of your walks and runs to be more difficult. As your body warms up, the effort will feel easier. Stick with it!

### *Pick a Pace*

After you warm up, gradually increase your speed until you hit a comfortable, steady pace. A good rule of thumb for moderate aerobic exercise is that your intensity should allow you to have a conversation without being out of breath.

### *Be Natural*

Let your body relax as you walk or run, using your natural stride length without overextending. Avoid tensing your hands, arms, and shoulders.

### *Find a Friend*

Doing your cardio program with a co-worker who is at a comparable level of fitness can provide a strong incentive to stay with your routine—being accountable to another person is a great way to keep you on track and make your sessions fly by as you get lost in conversation.

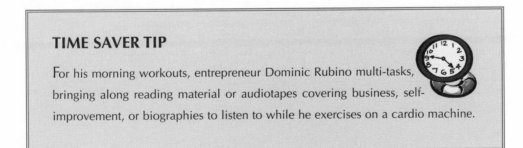

**TIME SAVER TIP**

For his morning workouts, entrepreneur Dominic Rubino multi-tasks, bringing along reading material or audiotapes covering business, self-improvement, or biographies to listen to while he exercises on a cardio machine.

### Stay Flexible

Use this workout plan as a guide, not a blueprint. As a business owner, your days are demanding and sometimes chaotic, with meetings, travel, and a hundred other things taking your time—so don't hesitate to change the workout days around to fit your schedule.

### Break it Up

Remember that research has found that two bouts of 15 minutes or three bouts of 10 minutes of exercise result in similar aerobic benefits to 30 continuous minutes of activity. And just 10 minutes of activity can boost mood and reduce fatigue. What's the bottom line? If you have to split your cardio into two daily sessions on a given day, or if you only have time for 10 minutes, just do it—don't use this as an excuse. For ideas on sneaking in cardio, see "Crafty Cardio."

## CRAFTY CARDIO

Here are some ways to sneak in activity during the day.

- Schedule walking meetings with your employees, or take longer phone calls on your cell phone or cordless and walk around the office or outside.

- Walk or jog around the baseball or soccer field during your child's practice or game.

- Walk to work, or park farther away from the office in the morning and after lunch.

- When you head out to get the mail or the newspaper, take a fast-paced walk around the block.

- Walk to lunch—and take a roundabout route to get there.

- At airports, walk the concourse while waiting for your flight—and don't take the "people mover" walkways.

### Don't Worry about Missing Workouts

If you skip a workout, it's not necessary to make it up the following day. And while it's typical to experience some tiredness when you begin a cardio routine, if you feel burned out, it's perfectly fine to repeat a given week before progressing on to the next. You've got enough competition and stress in your business life—cardio should be a break from that. So don't get caught up in the number of workouts you're doing or even in how much distance you can cover. Instead, focus on the joy of movement.

### Listen When Your Body's Talking

Learn to "listen to your body." While some muscle soreness after exercise is OK, if you feel joint pain or pain on one side of your body during a workout, stop and walk home. Wait until the pain dissipates before continuing your program, and head to your doctor if the pain continues.

### Think Safety

Be aware of your surroundings, and avoid wearing headphones when running near traffic. If you run at night, wear reflective gear and a light so you are visible to drivers.

### Keep Moving in Winter

Exercising in cold climates during winter can be a challenge—if weather is an issue where you live, exercise indoors on inclement days if you're not motivated to head outside or if the elements are too hazardous (when the temperature is 0 degrees Fahrenheit and wind speed is 15 mph, for example, frostbite can occur in 30 minutes). If you do go outside, keep it short and stay close to home for safety. Wear layers of clothing and look for material that is specially made to wick moisture and keep out rain and snow. If things warm up, you can take off unnecessary garments.

### The Next Step . . .

Looking beyond the three-month plan, and as you become fitter and fitter, you may want to add more cardio exercise days to your routine, run for longer times, or include interval and hill training (see "Taking It Up a Notch").

## IF YOU DON'T LIKE WALKING OR RUNNING

This cardio plan uses walking and running for aerobic exercise. These activities provide a good challenge to your cardiovascular system and are excellent ways to burn calories. But they are not, of course, the only ways to get your heart rate up. Claire Gruppo—founder and CEO of New York-based investment banking firm Gruppo, Levey & Co.—mixes up her cardio by biking and hiking in the summer and cross-country skiing in the winter. In the gym, she alternates among the stationary bike, treadmill, and stair stepper. "Actually, I find indoor cardio crushingly boring," she says. "So I read books while I'm on the machines." Other options include swimming and rowing. And if you prefer these, by all means do them. Or if you'd like to mix some of these pursuits with your walking and running, go right ahead.

You're much more likely to stick with a program if you like it—plus this type of "cross training" allows you to target a wide range of muscles. This helps you look better and prevent injuries due to muscle imbalances. "I have clients who are football players, and I put them on bikes and elliptical and rowing machines," NASM expert Robbins says. "Cross training is important because you're hitting different muscle groups, and the more variety the better."

Just keep in mind the principles of the cardio program—start very slowly, adding a little bit of total time (or distance) each week. And progress your workouts within a given week from easy to hard.

## WHICH GYM MACHINE IS BEST?

When it comes to improving your body's ability to use oxygen, cardio machines you find in health clubs or home gyms offer similar benefits. In a 2004 study published in the *Journal of Sports Medicine and Physical Fitness*, researchers assigned 22 moderately active women to one of three different types of cardio machines—a treadmill, elliptical trainer, and stair climber—and had participants work out three times a week. The women showed similar improvements in $VO_2$max, a measurement of how efficient the body is at using oxygen.

## TAKING IT UP A NOTCH

By the end of the three-month plan, you'll be ready to challenge yourself more by adding cardio sessions, increasing the length of workouts, and/or boosting intensity. Upping the intensity helps to prevent boredom and keeps your body from hitting a plateau that can result from doing the same routine time after time.

And there's another benefit—more fat loss. "By increasing the intensity, you're going to burn more calories from fat stores," Robbins says. "That's simply because you're burning more calories overall." And the extra work your body does, he adds, will boost your post-workout metabolism so that you burn even more calories when you're done with your session.

You should add intensity gradually, though, not pushing too hard. And remember to stay in the rotation discussed earlier: from easy to medium to hard days, and then back to low intensity. For this reason, the high-intensity workouts described in this section should be done only one day a week—on your hardest day.

So how do you raise the bar? By adding "intervals" or hills to your workouts. In fact, the final week of the three-month cardio program includes an optional interval/hills session to get you started.

To do intervals, simply intersperse harder running with easy running. Here's how it can look: After a 5- to 10-minute warm-up, run hard for 90 seconds, then easy for 90 seconds. You don't need to sprint, but just push to where it would be tough to hold a conversation. Repeat this one or two more times, then finish your run at your regular pace.

To run hills, find an incline of medium steepness that will take about a minute to run up. After a flat-ground warm-up, run up the hill at a steady pace, and walk or slowly jog back down. This is one "hill repeat." Repeat this one or two more times, and then finish your run on a flat surface.

As you progress, you can gradually add more intervals or hill repeats to the session. And you can add intensity with whatever type of cardio you're doing: on a bicycle, ride up and down hills; on a stationary bike, increase the tension for short bursts; on a treadmill, increase the speed or incline for brief periods. "It doesn't make a difference how you get your heart rate up," Robbins says. "You've just got to do something that will provide an overload."

## USING HEART RATE

It's not necessary to monitor your heart rate when doing aerobic activity, but doing so can help you more closely gauge your effort. You can pick up a basic heart-rate monitor for about $40 (visit www.polar-usa.us).

Generally, for moderate-intensity cardio, your heart rate should be about 65 percent of your maximum heart rate, which is estimated by using the formula of 220 minus your age. For the hard intervals, your heart rate should be 80 percent of your maximum heart rate. As an example, here are the numbers for a 40-year-old person:

Maximum heart rate = 220 – 40 = 180

65% of maximum heart rate = 180 x .65 = 117

80% of maximum heart rate = 180 x .80 = 144

### *Action* Items

➤ If you don't own running shoes, visit a local running store to purchase a pair.

➤ Although not mandatory, consider purchasing a sports watch this week.

➤ In the next several days, figure out a route that you can walk/run—keep it flat, if possible.

➤ Determine the best days and times of the week for you to do a cardio work out, and schedule three sessions for this week as you would business meetings. Leave at least a day between sessions. Do the same the following week (try to make the days and times consistent week to week).

## WORKOUT BOX

**Month 1**

*Week 1*

    Monday: Walk 10 minutes

    Wednesday: Walk 10 minutes

    Friday: Walk 10 minutes

*Week 2*

    Monday: Walk 10 minutes

    Wednesday: Walk 10 minutes

    Friday: Walk 12 minutes

*Week 3*

    Monday: Walk 10 minutes

    Wednesday: Walk 8 minutes, run 1 minute, walk 3 minutes (12 minutes total)

    Friday: Walk 5 minutes, run 2 minutes, repeat once (14 minutes)

*Week 4*

    Monday: Walk 15 minutes

    Wednesday: Walk 5 minutes, run 2 minutes, repeat once (14 minutes)

    Friday: Walk 4 minutes, run 2 minutes, repeat 2 twice (18 minutes)

**Month 2**

*Week 1*

    Monday: Walk 5 minutes, run 2 minutes, repeat once (14 minutes)

    Wednesday: Walk 4 minutes, run 2 minutes, repeat twice (18 minutes)

    Friday: Walk 3 minutes, run 2 minutes, repeat three times (20 minutes)

*Week 2*

    Monday: Walk 4 minutes, run 2 minutes, repeat twice (18 minutes)

    Wednesday: Walk 3 minutes, run 2 minutes, repeat three times (20 minutes)

    Friday: Walk 3 minutes, run 2½ minutes, repeat three times (22 minutes)

*Week 3*

> Monday: Walk 3 minutes, run 2 minutes, repeat three times (20 minutes)
>
> Wednesday: Walk 3 minutes, run 2½ minutes, repeat three times (22 minutes)
>
> Friday: Walk 3 minutes, run 3 minutes, repeat three times (24 minutes)

*Week 4*

> Monday: Walk 3 minutes, run 2½ minutes, repeat three times (22 minutes)
>
> Wednesday: Walk 3 minutes, run 3 minutes, repeat three times (24 minutes)
>
> Friday: Walk 2 minutes, run 3½ minutes, repeat four times (27½ minutes)

**Month 3**

*Week 1*

> Monday: Walk 3 minutes, run 3 minutes, repeat three times (24 minutes)
>
> Wednesday: Walk 2 minutes, run 3½ minutes, repeat four times (27½ minutes)
>
> Friday: Walk 2 minutes, run 4 minutes, repeat four times (30 minutes)

*Week 2*

> Monday: Walk 2 minutes, run 3½ minutes, repeat four times (27½ minutes)
>
> Wednesday: Walk 2 minutes, run 4 minutes, repeat four times (30 minutes)
>
> Friday: Walk 1 minute, run 5 minutes, repeat four times (30 minutes)

*Week 3*

> Monday: Walk 2 minutes, run 4 minutes, repeat four times (30 minutes)
>
> Wednesday: Walk 1 minute, run 5 minutes, repeat four times (30 minutes)
>
> Friday: Run 30 minutes

*Week 4*

> Monday: Walk 1 minute, run 5 minutes, repeat four times (30 minutes)
>
> Wednesday: Run 30 minutes
>
> Friday: Run 30 minutes (intervals/hills optional)

# CHAPTER 10

# Be Flexible

*I can really tell the difference when I don't have
stretching incorporated into my routine.*

—Entrepreneur Susan Solovic

## ONE-MINUTE SUMMARY

- Stretching is frequently neglected in fitness programs.
- That's a mistake, because flexibility exercises takes less time than you think and:
  - Help make everyday activities easier.
  - Allow you to maximize your other fitness pursuits.
  - Lessen muscle imbalances.
  - Provide a relaxing way to wind down from your exercise.
- Stretching shouldn't be competitive, and it shouldn't hurt.

> 🕐 Certain stretches will target particular muscle imbalances identified in the assessment in Chapter 4.
>
> 🕐 For extra credit, you can use a foam roller to target trigger points and relieve muscle knots.

Flexibility is one of the most underrated and overlooked aspects of fitness. Take a look in a typical health club, and you'll find a crowd in the weight room and on the treadmills. But you'll usually find plenty of space over in the stretching area.

And unfortunately, even those who do give flexibility exercises some attention often aren't going about it correctly. "A lot of people just don't know what they're doing or why they're doing it," says Tyler Wallace, director of clinical services for the NASM and a NASM corrective-exercise specialist. "The techniques many people are using just aren't proper."

## IT'S A STRETCH

So why does stretching get shortchanged? Well, at first glance, flexibility exercises may seem like an expendable part of your fitness routine. The results of good flexibility are more subtle than the visual effect of bigger muscles, so it's harder to appreciate the benefits. What's more, if you take the incorrect approach of "no pain, no gain" and you overdo a stretch, it can be pretty uncomfortable. "It shouldn't hurt, but when you take a stretch too far, it certainly can hurt," Wallace says.

Lastly, while some people are born with genetics that allow them to twist into circus-like contortions, many of us are not. So we may have long ago labeled ourselves as "inflexible"—setting up a mindset that trying to do anything about flexibility is just a waste of time.

But that's a mistake, Wallace says. "Flexibility should be as big a component [of fitness], if not more so, as everything else you're doing," he emphasizes. Here are just some of the reasons why you should make stretching part of your routine.

- Improving your flexibility has a practical application—it makes your everyday activities easier and may reduce injury risk. Pulling that book off the top shelf requires good mobility.
- If your muscles are tight, you won't be able to use them to their full potential and you'll sabotage your efforts in resistance training and cardio exercise. "Stretching gets your muscles to the right length so they can work properly as you reach for your other fitness goals," Wallace says.
- Staying flexible also may help lessen muscle imbalances and joint problems, which becomes more relevant as we spend more and more time sitting rather than putting our limbs and joints through their motions.
- Stretching doesn't require as much time as you think—you can have quick payoffs from minimal effort. In a study out of West Virginia University published in 2005, researchers found that stretching the hamstrings for just 30 seconds three times per week for four weeks was enough to increase the length of the muscle.
- Flexibility exercises after a workout offer a satisfying blend of the physiological and the psychological. Immediately following exercise, it takes a few minutes for your heart rate to come down, your perspiration to slow, and your breathing to ease. Your muscles are warm and relaxed. Using this time to stretch is a perfect way to bring a soothing calm as you enjoy the satisfaction that comes from exercise. Having just exerted yourself, the immediate lack of exertion feels that much sweeter. Soon you'll be back to the daily

## FLEXIBLE FACTS

"Flexibility" refers to your ability to move a joint or several joints through a full range of motion without pain. In general, women are more flexible than men, and the older we get the less flexible we tend to be—although this can be a result of inactivity and simply moving your joints less. And as strength can improve at older ages, so too can flexibility.

demands of your business, but for a few moments you can unwind and be in the moment.

Getting started is easy. In fact, if you've included the stretches from the Quick-Start Action Plan, you've already begun reaping benefits. This chapter provides a few more straightforward stretches to keep you on the fast track to better flexibility.

## THE FLEXIBILITY PROGRAM

Here are some ground rules before you get going with your flexibility program.

- *Be sane about pain.* Remember: stretching should not be painful. If it is, you're asking for an injury. At most, you should move to a position of mild tension. If you feel any sharp pains, ease back on the stretch or just release it altogether. If you have any special issues—knee problems, for example—use caution. Don't have a predetermined notion of how far you should be able to stretch. Everyone is different, so work within your boundaries.
- *Relax.* Focus on keeping your whole body in a relaxed state during your stretches. Have your jaw, shoulders, feet, and hands stay loose, and keep breathing throughout the entire stretch.
- *Stay put.* Hold each stretch end point for 15 to 30 seconds, and don't bounce.
- *Draw in.* While you perform each exercise, do the "drawing-in" maneuver you learned about in Chapter 2—pulling the belly button in toward the spine.
- *Fix imbalances.* In Chapter 4, you pinpointed muscle imbalances you may have with the NASM Overhead Squat Assessment. Take a moment to look at your self-assessment results on pages 61–62. Included with this chapter's

### TIME SAVER TIP

If you belong to a gym, ask if they have half-hour training sessions with trainers rather than the usual hour sessions. (For more on how to pick a gym and trainer, see Chapter 14.)

## GOING THE DISTANCE

For Mike Nagel, stretching is an important part of his training routine. And for good reason—he's a triathlete competing in Ironman® races that involve a 2.4-mile swim, a 112-mile bike ride, and a 26.2-mile marathon run—done back-to-back-to-back. When training for those kinds of distances, his muscles take punishment. "If I have some muscles that are sore, like the calves or Achilles tendon or hips," he says, "I'll get up from my desk and do stretches during the day." He also is a big believer in massage therapy, he adds, and gets a massage every two weeks. "I find it keeps me away from those nagging injuries."

His intense training routine helps him stay alert, organized, and energetic on the job, says Nagel, co-founder of Vascular Solutions Inc. (In 2005, he took on a new challenge as vice president of sales and marketing at Incisive Surgical, a start-up company that features an absorbable surgical staple.) To help make his training a more seamless part of his life, his wife often joins him in exercise. "She'll do part of the long runs with me," he says. "For some of my recovery bike rides, where I go a little bit slower, we'll ride together."

During his youth, Nagel struggled with his weight and says, even to this day, that serves as a motivation for him to stay physically fit. And the grueling Ironman®, he believes, has a lesson to teach the entrepreneur. "You just take it one step at a time," he explains, "and sometimes you have to dig deep, and you have to think of ways to succeed and get through. Failure is not an option. There's no magic to it."

And in the end, while finishing the race is a thrill, the hard work and discipline it takes to get there are where the real satisfaction lies. "It's just like building a company," Nagel says. "It's the journey along the way that is the most fun."

description of the stretches is an indication of which muscle imbalance checkpoints a particular stretch will help address. It's especially important to include those exercises that will target your particular imbalances. After

---

## CAT STRETCH FEVER

Cats are good role models when it comes to flexibility. They stretch after they wake up, before they eat, and in between their 15 daily naps. They stretch whenever the mood strikes, and not as part of some predetermined schedule (cats don't have schedules). So be catlike and incorporate some stretches into your day just for the fun of it.

---

four or six weeks, you should see significant improvement in the Overhead Squat Assessment.

- *Save it for last.* Aim to include stretching after your cardio workout, when the muscles are warmer, circulation is increased, and joints are more limber. (Instead of stretching *before* exercising, simply warm up by going at a very easy pace to gradually get your body adapted.) Also, keep in mind that you can take quick stretching breaks at any time and wherever it's convenient—in your office, at home, in a hotel room, or waiting in the airport.

### THE STRETCHES

Perform these stretches at least two days a week, doing one rep per leg or side, and one set per stretch. Remember to hold each move for 15 to 30 seconds. All photos are courtesy of Karen Thomas of Entrepreneur Press and photographer Julia Cappelli.

FORWARD LEAN
*Muscles stretched*: Calf
*Targets imbalances around the feet*
This is a two-part stretch. Face a wall or stable object with your feet a little less than shoulder-width apart and pointed straight ahead. Step toward the wall with one foot, and lean forward to place your hands

FIGURE 10.1: **Forward Lean**

A. Back Leg Straight

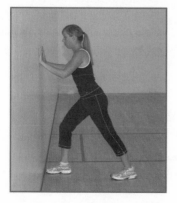

against the wall. With your back leg straight, lower your back heel toward the floor to feel a stretch in your back leg. Gently lean farther into the wall to apply more tension and hold (see Figure 10.1A). For the next part of the stretch, slightly bend your back leg and hold (see Figure 10.1B). Repeat the sequence with the opposite leg.

FIGURE 10.1: **Forward Lean**

B. Back Leg Bent

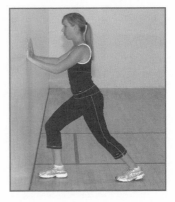

LYING STRAIGHT LEG STRETCH

*Muscles stretched*: Hamstrings (the back of your thighs)

*Targets imbalances around the knees and low back*

Lie on your back with your legs bent and feet flat on the floor. Holding both ends of a towel or cord, wrap this around the bottom of one foot and straighten the leg (see Figure 10.2A). Keeping your foot flexed, gently lift your leg until you feel a slight stretch in the back of your thigh, and hold (see Figure 10.2B). Repeat with the opposite leg.

FIGURE 10.2: **Lying Straight Leg Stretch**

A. Start

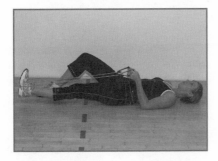

B. Movement

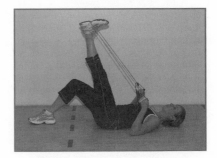

---

## SWEATIN' IT OUT

If you're out of shape, you may think you'll sweat more when you work out. But generally that's not the case. As you get in better shape, your rate of perspiration increases. This is because sweating is your body's way of cooling itself—as sweat evaporates, it takes body heat with it. When you exercise regularly, the body adapts and learns to get better at cooling itself by boosting your sweat output.

KNEEL AND REACH STRETCH

*Muscles stretched*: Hips, quadriceps (the front of your thighs), back

*Targets imbalances around the low back and shoulders*

Kneel on the ground, with your left knee forward and bent to 90 degrees, and your hands on your hips. Gently lean your body forward from the hips to feel a slight stretch in your right hip and the front of your thigh. Next, lift your right arm overhead (see Figure 10.3A) and toward the left (see Figure 10.3B), and hold. Return to start and repeat with right leg forward. Avoid this stretch if you have any knee problems.

FIGURE 10.3: **Kneel and Reach Stretch**

A. Start

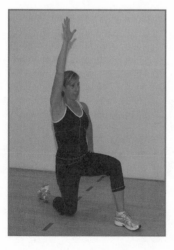

B. Movement

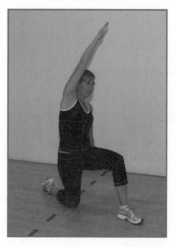

SIDE-TO-SIDE STRETCH

*Muscles stretched*: Inner thigh

*Targets imbalances around the knees*

Stand with your feet wide apart and toes pointed straight ahead (see Figure 10.4A). Bend your right knee slightly, gently shift your weight toward the right (see Figure 10.4B), and hold. You'll feel a stretch in the left inner thigh. Repeat with left knee bent.

FIGURE 10.4: **Side-to-Side Stretch**

A. Start

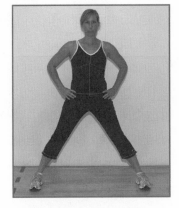

B. Movement

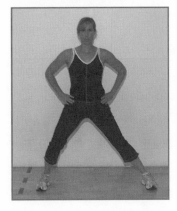

BACK STRETCH

*Muscles stretched*: Back and shoulder

*Targets imbalances around the shoulders*

Kneel on all fours directly in front of a chair or another object of similar height (pictured is a stability exercise ball). Place your left arm on the chair, with your arm straight and thumb up. Lower your torso to feel a gentle stretch and hold (see Figure 10.5). Repeat with your right hand on the chair.

FIGURE 10.5: **Back Stretch**

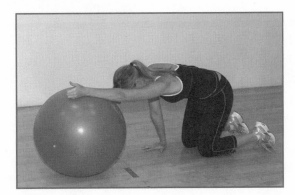

FIGURE 10.6: **Chest Stretch**

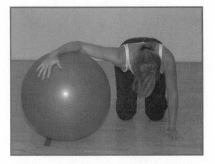

CHEST STRETCH

*Muscles stretched*: Chest

*Targets imbalances around the shoulders*

Kneel on all fours next to a chair or another object of similar height (pictured is a stability exercise ball). Bend your elbow to 90 degrees and lift your arm straight out to the side, resting your elbow on the chair. Gently lower your torso to feel a slight stretch in your chest and front shoulder area, and hold (see Figure 10.6). Repeat with opposite arm. You can also do this exercise while standing in a doorway—with your elbow bent to 90 degrees, place your arm against the wall near the door frame, and gently lean forward.

FIGURE 10.7: **Neck Stretch**

A. Looking up

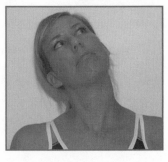

B. Looking down

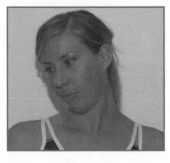

NECK STRETCH

*Muscles stretched*: Neck

*Targets imbalance in head movement*

While standing or sitting, tilt your head to the right, feeling a light stretch on the left side, and hold. Rotate your head upward so that you're looking toward the ceiling (see Figure 10.7A) and hold. Return to the start. Next, tilt your head to the right again, then rotate your head downward (see Figure 10.7B) and hold. Repeat this entire sequence to the left side. Don't tilt your head straight back—this can overstress your upper spine.

## EXTRA CREDIT

If you've ever felt a knot in a muscle, you've probably experienced something called a "trigger point." This knot occurs where a specific part of the muscle becomes shortened and taut, and may be caused by microtraumas brought on over time by inactivity, bad posture, vitamin deficiencies, and joint abnormalities. Even something like propping a telephone between your shoulder and ear or using a chair with inadequate back support can cause trigger points.

Although this often doesn't cause any pain unless you compress the area, a trigger point can lead to muscle weakness and stiffness, and may limit your movement. It's been referred to as the "weakest link" in your muscle chain.

The good news is you can do something to help alleviate trigger points. By using self-massage to apply light pressure to a knot, you'll prompt the muscle fibers to realign properly and return to their normal length.

To target your trigger points, NASM recommends using a foam roller to self-massage your muscles—this is a six-inch round, foot-long piece of foam that you place your body weight on and roll along your muscle. You can pick up a roller for less than $10 through Perform Better at www.performbetter.com. (Another option is a device with handles called The Stick®, which you roll crossways against your muscles—visit www.thestick.com). Once you roll onto a tender spot, you've found a trigger point, and you should keep light pressure on the site for at least 20 or 30

### A HISTORY OF BACK PROBLEMS

The concept of trigger points actually has played a role in U.S. history. In the 1950s, one of the pioneers in the understanding of trigger points, Janet G. Travell, M.D., successfully treated John F. Kennedy's chronic back problems by injecting an anesthetic drug into trigger points in his back (she also adjusted for his shorter left leg by having him wear a heel lift). The success of the treatment reportedly enabled JFK—who previously was having difficulty even walking—to run for the White House. Travell later went on to become Kennedy's personal physician during his presidency.

seconds. Be warned—this can be uncomfortable, but realize that the payoff is better flexibility and your muscles performing at their max.

You can do these "extra credit" stretches before your other stretches when you cool down from your cardio. Try to fit one or more of them in if you can—you'll make your knots not a problem! Keep your abdominals drawn in and tighten your glutes. And if you have back or joint problems, consult with your physician first.

FIGURE 10.8: **Calf Stretch with Foam Roller**

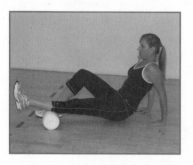

CALF STRETCH WITH FOAM ROLLER
*Targets imbalances around the feet*
Sit on the ground with your legs straight out in front of you, and use your hands to prop yourself up. Position the foam roller under your calf, and then roll from the lower portion of the calf until you find a tender area (see Figure 10.8). Hold the position, waiting until the soreness diminishes significantly. Move on and find another tender area and repeat. Then switch to the opposite leg. (Keep one leg crossed over the other during the exercise for added pressure.)

FIGURE 10.9: **Hamstrings Stretch with Foam Roller**

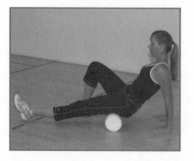

HAMSTRINGS STRETCH WITH FOAM ROLLER
*Targets imbalances around the knees and low back*
Again sitting with your legs out in front and using your hands to prop yourself up, position the foam roller under the back of your thigh (see Figure 10.9). Roll from the knee area toward your hip until you find a tender area. Hold the position, waiting until the soreness diminishes significantly. Move on and find another tender area and repeat. Repeat with the opposite leg. (Keep one leg crossed over the other during the exercise for added pressure.)

QUADRICEPS STRETCH WITH FOAM ROLLER

*Targets imbalances around the low back*

FIGURE 10.10: **Quadriceps Stretch with Foam Roller**

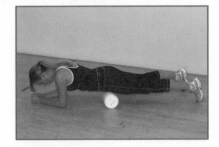

Lie face down with the foam roller under your thigh, and your upper body propped up on your elbows. Roll your thigh from the hip area toward the knee until you find a tender area (see Figure 10.10). Hold the position, waiting until the soreness diminishes significantly. Move on and find another tender area and repeat. Repeat with the opposite leg.

---

### *Action* Items

➤ If you've been reluctant to try stretching in the past, take a minute to think about why. Was it a matter of not having enough time? Or were you just resigned to the idea that you weren't flexible so it wouldn't help?

➤ Review how you did in the NASM Overhead Squat Assessment in Chapter 4. Did you notice any particular muscle imbalances?

➤ After two of your cardio sessions this week, include at least three of the stretches from this chapter, focusing on any muscle imbalances you may have. As you progress, add more stretches.

---

# WORKOUT BOX

**Stretches**

| Exercise | Repetitions | Sets |
|---|---|---|
| Forward lean | 1 | 1 |
| Lying straight leg stretch | 1 | 1 |
| Kneel and reach stretch | 1 | 1 |
| Side-to-side stretch | 1 | 1 |
| Back stretch | 1 | 1 |
| Chest stretch | 1 | 1 |
| Neck stretch | 1 | 1 |

**Extra Credit**

| Exercise | Repetitions | Sets |
|---|---|---|
| Calf stretch with foam roller | 1 | 1 |
| Hamstrings stretch with foam roller | 1 | 1 |
| Quadriceps stretch with foam roller | 1 | 1 |

# PART IV

# *Guaranteeing Your Return on Investment*

# CHAPTER 11

# More Energy,
# Less Stress

*I was eating poorly and not sleeping enough. That's just a bad combination. Now I'm making sure I get seven and a half hours of sleep a night and eating healthy, and I have a lot more energy. I feel a lot better about myself, and when you feel better about yourself, you're able to better serve your clients.*

—JON LIEB, FOUNDER AND MANAGING DIRECTOR OF THIRTY INK MEDIA & MARKETING

## ONE-MINUTE SUMMARY

🕐 Chronic stress can lead to illness, negative thinking, and a lack of energy.

🕐 You can help control stress and increase energy by focusing on four core elements of your day: sleep, food, movement, and awareness.

🕐 Sleep strategies include watching your caffeine intake (for some people, caffeine even 12 hours before bedtime can disrupt sleep), taking a 15- to 20-minute power nap just after noontime and before the postlunch "dip," and exercising in the early evening.

- Fatty foods make you sluggish, while protein sources such as lean poultry increase alertness—adding extra at lunch can help perk you up for an afternoon meeting.
- In addition to physical benefits, yoga's movements can boost your energy and mood, and decrease stress.
- Relaxation techniques increase awareness—which translates into reduced stress, better concentration, energy, and productivity.

Stress is so pervasive in our society that we take it to be an inevitable part of surviving the day-to-day challenges we face. And when you're starting and growing a business, going through intensely stressful times has become a right of passage.

The trouble is, chronic stress works silently to sabotage your efforts to eat well, get fit, and stay healthy so you can be there for your business, family, and friends. Constant elevated levels of the stress hormone cortisol can boost your appetite and add extra pounds, as well as increase your chances of depression, heart disease, and other illnesses. In fact, almost two-thirds of the ailments doctors see in their offices result from stress, according to the Society for Neuroscience, a group of more than 37,000 scientists and physicians involved in studying the brain and nervous system. To make matters worse, the "fight or flee" response that stress induces tends to foster negative thinking that undermines the optimism and enthusiasm your business requires.

At the same time that we feel overburdened by stress, we can feel a dearth of energy. Stress is yin to energy's yang, robbing you of vitality and inner resources you need at work and in the rest of your life. When stress becomes pervasive, it takes the joy out of living.

But by focusing on four core elements of your day—sleep, food, movement, and awareness—you can improve your ability to manage stress and maximize your energy. Each of these has a profound effect on body and mind, and each provides a foundation on which you can build a vigorous life, putting you in control of how you react to the constant challenges you face as an entrepreneur.

## STRESS FALLOUT

According to the U.S. Department of Health and Human Services, stress can contribute to:

- Sleep problems
- Headaches
- Constipation
- Diarrhea
- Irritability
- Poor energy and concentration
- Eating excessively

- Weight gain or loss
- Heart problems and high blood pressure
- Diabetes
- Neck and back pain
- Difficulty getting pregnant
- Anger
- Stomach cramping

### SLEEP

Getting sufficient shut-eye is important to your ability to manage daily stress, problem solve, and stay energized for your work. "People think that sleep is negotiable," says Mark Mahowald, M.D., a Minneapolis, Minnesota-based neurologist quoted in *Sleepmatters*, the newsletter of the National Sleep Foundation (www.sleepfoundation.org). "They wear sleep deprivation as a badge of honor. Have you ever noticed that no one brags about how much sleep they get?" But, Mahowald says, sleep is as important as eating, drinking, or exercise.

However, it's easy to fall into the trap of thinking sleep is expendable when the demands of business are high—and it may seem that you're actually getting by on a short-term basis. Even someone who goes without a night of sleep can stay alert for interesting and challenging tasks, says sleep expert Chris Idzikowski, Ph.D., who consults with British Airways on helping passengers handle jet lag and is the director of the Edinburgh Sleep Centre in Scotland. But if you're in a less invigorating environment, the effects of poor sleep could show up at the worst time—such as at a meeting with a monotonous speaker. "With that kind of dull environment," Idzikowski says, "the danger of falling asleep in the meeting suddenly becomes high."

## SLEEP AND BANKRUPTCY?

The effects of a poor night of sleep can be so subtle you may not even notice them. That's because sleep loss affects the prefrontal cortex, which is the area of the brain involved in higher-order thinking, such as judgment and making decisions. In a 2000 study conducted at Loughborough University in the United Kingdom, researchers had people play a business simulation game. Before playing, some of the players had gone without sleep for 36 hours (essentially missing a night of sleep), and others had been allowed to sleep. The demands of the game became increasingly difficult, and the players had to sell a product in a highly competitive market. The sleep-deprived participants persisted in applying solutions that had worked earlier but were no longer useful. Instead of innovation, it seems, they relied on futile repetition. The results: they either went bankrupt or came close to it. Subjects who weren't sleep deprived did fine.

What's more, when you don't get enough sleep, you begin to build up a "sleep debt." The more sleep you miss, the more debt you accumulate, and the greater your tendency to feel sleepy. "It's almost like holding one's breath," Idzikowski says. "You can [go with inadequate sleep] for a while, but you can't do it forever." In fact, missing out on two or three hours of sleep at night for just a week reduces alertness, performance, and mood. And as your fatigue increases, you may be susceptible to greater risk-taking behavior. Recent research also is showing that sleep deprivation may be associated with chronic disease, including diabetes and heart disease, according to the *Tufts University Health & Nutrition Letter.*

The amount of sleep needed varies by individual—as a general guide, most adults require between seven and nine hours of downtime, according to the National Sleep Foundation. Some people can feel fine with just six hours, while others need ten. Jeff Bezos, founder of Amazon.com, and Netscape Communications Corporation co-founder Marc Andreessen reportedly both sleep for eight hours a night. "I am not any good on less than six hours sleep," says Claire Gruppo, who runs the investment-banking firm Gruppo, Levey & Co. "I try to sleep seven. And I think it's a very, very rare human being who can function supremely well on less than that."

How do you know if you're getting enough sleep? If you find it difficult to keep alert when sitting through a particularly boring or monotonous meeting, it's a sign that you may not be allowing yourself sufficient good-quality sleep. Other indications include being irritable with your employees, family, or friends, and having trouble focusing or recalling facts—an obvious detriment to your business. To help yourself to better slumber, here are some sleep-friendly tips to keep in mind.

> *There is plenty of compelling evidence supporting the argument that sleep is the most important predictor of how long you will live, perhaps more important than whether you smoke, exercise, or have high blood pressure or cholesterol levels.*
>
> —WILLIAM DEMENT, M.D., FROM HIS BOOK *THE PROMISE OF SLEEP* (DELL, 2000)

### Be Caffeine Conscious

Some people have trouble getting to sleep up to 12 hours after even a small serving of caffeine. If you're having difficulty sleeping and you're in the habit of an afternoon cup of coffee, try cutting down on coffee and other caffeine-containing drinks and foods after noontime for two weeks to see if it helps your sleep. While having two 8-ounce cups of caffeinated beverage a day is considered a moderate intake, be aware that kitchen mugs can hold 10 ounces and travel mugs 16 ounces.

### Avoid Alcohol before Bedtime

It's tempting to think that a glass of wine or a beer is a good way to unwind before bed. But drinking within 60 minutes of bedtime appears to interfere with the second half of sleep time as the effects of the alcohol wear off (some research even indicates that moderately imbibing six hours before hitting the sack can cause sleep troubles). That interrupted shuteye means you'll be dragging the next day. If you overdo it on a given night, you can help alleviate the dehydrating effects of alcohol by drinking a glass of water before bed for each drink you had.

### Power Nap

Most of us feel an energy lull in the afternoons. Although this is known as the postlunch "dip," the characteristic sleepiness can happen whether or not you eat lunch, explain Michael Smolensky, Ph.D., and Lynne Lamberg in *The Body Clock*

## STRESSED ON THE JOB

A survey reported in 2006 and done by Day-Timers Inc. (a manufacturer of organizational products) found that compared with a decade earlier, U.S. workers are inundated with e-mail (an average of 46 a day), voice mail, and cell phone calls. In 1994, the average time sitting in front of the work computer was 9.5 hours per week. Now it's nearly 16 hours.

*Guide to Better Health* (Henry Holt and Company, 2000). Natural circadian rhythms probably play a role, and some of us experience a bigger drain than others. If your schedule allows, try to fit in a 15 to 20 minute nap during the day. It's easier to do if you work out of your home, obviously, but try it even if you're in an office—close your door or go to your car. The best time to squeeze in some rest seems to be after lunch but before the "dip" kicks in. Japanese researchers found that when test subjects grabbed 20 minutes of Z's just after noontime, they reported being less sleepy and better at task performance during the rest of the day.

### Exercise

With an early evening workout session, your body temperature rises—and that's followed with a temperature drop later in the evening, which encourages sleep. But keep in mind that if you exercise too close to bedtime—within three hours—you may experience more difficulty sleeping because your body temperature is still elevated. Also, remember that it's best to exercise during the time of day when it fits with your schedule and when you feel the most motivated—making it more likely that you'll follow through.

### Enjoy a Warm Shower

Hopping into a warm shower or bath about an hour and a half before bedtime not only relaxes tense muscles, it prompts a body temperature decrease after you get out, making your body primed for sleep.

### *Keep a Schedule*

Try to stick to about the same times for going to bed and waking up, even on weekends. This will help trigger a consistent fall in body temperature around bedtime. This can be a challenge when traveling—see Chapter 12 for tips on dealing with the effects of jet lag.

### *Clean Up Your Environment*

Don't use your bedroom for work, if possible. Most experts say that keeping your room slightly cool fosters good sleep, and try to minimize random outside noise—a fan, a waterfall CD, or other "white noise" can help mask disruptions. The web site www.sleepmachines.com has background noises for seemingly every taste—rain, wind, and beach sounds, but also sounds of the furnace and, believe it or not, the dishwasher.

### *Seek Help*

If you have problems with sleep for more than a week, talk to your doctor. He or she may recommend medication or suggest that you see a sleep specialist. Consistent trouble with getting to sleep or awaking too early may be a signal of mild depression.

---

## SLEEP AND OBESITY

Poor sleep habits can have a direct effect on your waistline, according to a 2004 study by Columbia University researchers. They found an association between obesity risk and how many hours people slept each night. People who snoozed four or fewer hours had a 73 percent greater chance of obesity than those who managed to get between seven and nine hours of shuteye. People who slept six hours a night had a 23 percent increased risk of being significantly overweight. One explanation may be that insufficient sleep decreases the hormone leptin, which plays a role in regulating appetite.

---

## FOOD

Your food choices can influence your energy and stress. Sugary snacks, for example, wreak havoc by spiking blood sugar levels, which then drop quickly and send you into a tailspin of fatigue. But sugar isn't the only food to watch for.

### *Forgo Fatty Foods*

A high-fat meal can leave you feeling lethargic because it tends to park in the stomach, diverting blood from muscles and vital organs—including your brain. Fat also makes the blood thicker and less efficient at delivering oxygen—leaving you less able to manage a stressful situation.

By following the Entrepreneur Diet (which includes smart fast-food choices), you'll ensure you're not filling up on too much fat. But if you tend to fall back on fatty fast food, take a few minutes to check out the nutrition information on the web sites of the restaurants you frequent to get an idea which items are the lowest in fat, or ask for a nutrition fact sheet at the counter. In addition to the fast-food and restaurant options in the Entrepreneur Diet, Figure 11.1 shows some more

### TIME SAVER TIP

If you enjoy cooking but not all the hassles of grocery shopping and cleanup, try a meal prep kitchen. A number of businesses (with franchise opportunities) have popped up recently to help make your meal preparation as easy as possible. They do the food shopping, food prep, and recipe planning ahead of time, and you show up at their location to assemble the food into 6 to 12 meals (with about four servings per meal), which takes a couple of hours. You bring home the meals, freeze, and serve in the days ahead. For more information, visit www.dreamdinners.com, www.mygirlfriendskitchen.com, www.dinnerbydesign.com, www.supersuppers.com, or www.supperthymeusa.com.

examples of ways you can cut down the fat. Notice that what you may have assumed is healthy—chicken salad and tuna—are big-calorie items.

### Munch on Magnesium

Magnesium is a mineral that plays a role in bone strength and heart rhythm. What's more, research indicates that if you're low on magnesium, while exercising

FIGURE 11.1: **Making Better Choices**

| Instead of this . . . | Try this . . . |
|---|---|
| Burger King® Double Whopper with cheese (990 calories, 64 grams fat) | Burger King® BK Veggie Burger, no mayo (340 calories, 8 grams fat) |
| Arby's® Chicken Salad Sandwich (880 calories, 45 grams fat) | Arby's® Hot Ham & Swiss Melt (270 calories, 8 grams fat) |
| Pizza Hut® 14-inch Large Stuffed Crust Meat Lover's Pizza (450 calories, 21 grams fat for one slice) | Pizza Hut® 14-inch Fit n' Delicious Pizza™ Green Pepper, Red Onion & Diced Red Tomato (140 calories, 4 grams fat for one slice) |
| Jack in the Box® Bacon Ultimate Cheeseburger (1,090 calories, 77 grams fat) | Jack in the Box® Chicken Caesar Salad with Reduced Fat Herb Mayo Dressing (269 calories, 12 grams of fat) |
| Kentucky Fried Chicken® Double Crunch Sandwich (530 calories, 28 grams fat) | Kentucky Fried Chicken® Tender Roast Sandwich without sauce (260 calories, 5 grams fat) |
| Church's® Chicken Spicy Thigh (one piece) with Sweet Corn Nuggets (1,080 calories, 64 grams fat) | Church's® Original Breast (two pieces) with Collard Greens (425 calories, 22 grams fat) |
| Subway® 6-inch Tuna Sandwich (530 calories, 31 grams fat) | Subway® 6-inch Turkey Breast Sandwich with 1 T. Light Mayo (330 calories, 10 grams fat) |

> *I try to eat as much protein during the day as I can. It seems to keep me constant on my energy.*
> —Max Hoes, co-owner and co-founder of CFR Line

your body uses up more oxygen and your heart beats faster. Bottom line: you fatigue faster. And yet, according to the U.S. Department of Agriculture's Agricultural Research Service, just 32 percent of Americans get the recommended daily amounts of this nutrient—420 mg for men older than age 30 and 320 mg for women older than age 30 (amounts differ for pregnant or nursing women).

You can boost your magnesium intake by snacking on soybeans, pumpkin seeds, trail mix, and low-fat vanilla yogurt. Other sources include garbanzo beans, lima beans, bran muffins, and spinach.

## Perk Up with Protein

Protein appears to increase alertness by boosting an energy-enhancing brain chemical called dopamine. On the other hand, carbohydrates tend to make us more calm and sleepy by raising the brain's level of serotonin.

If you're eating soon before a business meeting or you need to sit down and work on a project for an extended time, add extra protein to the meal (such as lean chicken or pork) and go lighter on the carbohydrates (such as breads and pastas). For example, if you visit Subway for a chicken breast sandwich, ask for an extra amount of chicken.

### RHODIOLA ROSEA

This herb, known as an "adaptogen" for its purported ability to return the body to proper balance, may play a role in combating stress, which can upset hormonal balance. It also may benefit the heart and slightly delay muscle fatigue during exercise. When *Rhodiola rosea* was given to rats, they boosted the time they could swim before exhaustion by 24.6 percent. Look for *Rhodiola rosea L.* root extract (a typical daily dosage is 100 to 600 mg a day for 1½ to 3 months), but check with your doctor before supplementing.

## THE STRESS RESPONSE

When confronted with a perceived threat, the body releases stress hormones, such as epinephrine (also known as adrenaline) and cortisol. These chemicals help you become more focused and stronger, as well as to react faster. This so-called "fight or flee" response is a good thing in the short term if a tiger is chasing you, but it isn't so good when you face traffic jams, demanding clients, and other modern pressures that provide a steady flow of stress. When stress lingers and becomes chronic, your body remains in a heightened state of alert. In effect, instead of sharper peaks of stress followed by valleys of relaxation and recovery, we experience an endless series of stress hills, with little break between. So now, the same stress response that was helpful for short-term survival is throwing a wrench in your body's finely tuned biochemical system.

## MOVEMENT

While vigorous exercise can be an excellent way to blow off steam and increase your energy, there are also stress and energy benefits from movement that is more deliberate and slow. Allowing your mind to concentrate on precisely controlling your body provides the perfect distraction from the intrusive thoughts of your business concerns. One of the best ways to do this is with the practice of yoga.

Yoga has been around for more than 5,000 years, having originated in India, and has been growing in popularity in the United States. Even pro athletes have taken it up. The practice has great physical benefits—reducing soreness after a new exercise routine, for example. Yoga also has proved helpful in decreasing low back pain and pain from osteoarthritis in the hands, and may help control cardiovascular disease and insulin resistance (which can lead to diabetes).

In addition, yoga can boost your energy and mood, as well as decrease stress. In a 2005 study published in the journal *Medical Science Monitor*, researchers looked at the effects of yoga on a group of women who reported feeling emotionally distressed. After 12 weeks of yoga done for 90 minutes at least twice a week, the women said they had significantly reduced stress compared with a

## THE YOGA PATH

Nancy LeClaire, who operates a sole-proprietor business training people to become certified financial planners, practices yoga between five and seven days a week, and says she enjoys the variety yoga brings to her exercise routine. "I was not flexible at all when I started doing yoga," she recalls. "I couldn't touch my toes." She's come a long way—she recently became a registered instructor and, in her off hours, teaches yoga to seniors in her community.

An accountant by training, LeClaire has worked at CPA firms, but prefers having her own consulting business. "I like the flexibility," she says, "and I didn't like the restrictions of working for a corporation."

One of the keys to entrepreneurial success, she says, is being able to sell yourself. "I'm not afraid to tell people that I can do a good job, because I wouldn't do something unless I thought I could."

Yoga has helped LeClaire become happier, less prone to worry, and more open to change, she says. "In yoga, as your body becomes more flexible and as you listen to some of the words said in class, your mind also becomes a little bit more open," she explains. "Yoga has changed my life." She's even found a way to combine yoga with her entrepreneurial spirit by developing a product called the "yoga stick," and a corresponding workshop to help ease shoulder tension.

To get started with yoga, LeClaire recommends checking out the local YMCA or college for introductory yoga classes. Yoga studios tend to be a little more expensive, she adds, costing upward of $100 a month or around $10 per class. Another option is working with a private teacher who can show you how to develop a practice you can do at home.

nonyoga group, and yogis also showed significant improvement in scores of vigor, fatigue, depression, and well-being. In another study, published in 1992 and conducted at Brooklyn College, City University of New York, yoga was found to be at least as effective as swimming in reducing measures of tension, fatigue, and anger in college students. One possible reason: yoga appears to reduce levels of the stress hormone cortisol.

If you have time to try a yoga class, you may find the structured setting is a good way to keep up your routine. Some instructors will offer a mixture of different styles. Ask ahead of time about the pacing of the class and how long you'll have to hold the poses. If you'll be performing meditation or chanting, this indicates the session will be more contemplative and less strenuous.

You can still incorporate yoga into your day if you don't have time for a class. Try some postures at the end of your workouts or as part of a daily work break. "You can do yoga at night before you go to bed," suggests entrepreneur Margaret Moore, who has successfully launched two companies in the past ten years. "That's easy to fit in, and it's a nice way to unwind." Use a quiet room without any distractions. As you perform each posture, focus on your breathing to bring a greater sense of calm to your mind and body. Here are some postures to get you started—for more postures, *Yoga* (Sterling Publishing Co., Inc., 2002) by Liz Lark is a helpful and easy-to-follow source.

## Yoga Exercises

### CAT STRETCH

Get on all fours, with your hands beneath your shoulders, your back straight, and your neck in line with your spine. As you inhale, slowly arch your back and look up, holding the position for a few breaths. Next, as you exhale let your head slowly drop down and round your back (as a "stretching" feline would). Hold for a few breaths, then repeat this sequence between one and three more times.

### TWIST

Lie on your back, legs straight. With both hands, pull your right knee toward your chest, grasping below the knee. Next release your right hand to the floor and lower the right knee to your left side, gently pulling the knee toward the floor with your left hand. Make sure your shoulders remain flat on the ground so that you rotate from the hips (keeping your right arm straight out to the side will help). Rotate your head gently to the right. Hold for a few breaths and then return to the starting position. Repeat with your left leg. Avoid this exercise if you have back, hip, or knee problems.

THE WARRIOR

Standing with your feet together, spread your legs wide and extend your arms straight out to your sides, parallel to the ground. Turn your right foot out and then bend your right knee to no more than a 90-degree angle, keeping your arms parallel to the ground and at shoulder level. Hold for a few breaths and then return to the beginning position. Repeat on the left side.

## AWARENESS

You can spend so much of your day solving problems and meeting the needs of others—customers, family, friends—that your focus is nearly always external. Especially for the fast-paced days (and nights) of an entrepreneur, there doesn't seem to be time to slow down, stop, and turn the mind's attention to your own inner world. In *The Anxiety & Phobia Workbook, 3rd Edition* (New Harbinger Publications, 2000)—an excellent source for dealing with anxiety and panic—Edmund J. Bourne, Ph.D., points out that we almost never "experience ourselves 'just being' in the present moment. For many people in Western society, in fact, the idea of doing nothing or 'just being' is difficult to comprehend."

By practicing relaxation techniques, you can accomplish this increased awareness of your own being—an awareness of yourself separate and apart from the demands of your business and other responsibilities. Before you start thinking this is getting a little too "touchy feely" and better left to monastery-dwelling monks, realize that there are concrete benefits to you, your business, and everyone around you: reduced stress and better concentration, energy, and productivity. Writes Bourne: "Even sleep can fail to break the cumulative stress cycle unless you've given yourself permission to deeply relax while awake."

Each of the following awareness techniques (described in Bourne's *Workbook*) can be practiced just about anywhere at any time in as little as five or ten minutes. It's best to use a place that is quiet without distractions, but make do where you can—in the office, at home, on a plane. And the more you practice, the easier and faster it will be to achieve a relaxed state.

## *Deep Breathing*

Without realizing it, your breathing can often become shallow, emanating from the chest rather than the abdomen, especially when you are anxious. Focusing on deeper breathing from the belly helps induce a feeling of relaxation, and may even help lower blood pressure.

How to Do It

- Sitting in a comfortable chair or lying down, place one hand slightly above your belly button.
- Take a slow, deep breath through your nose, feeling as though you're filling every part of your lungs.
- Your hand should be pushed out as your belly expands.
- Pause for a second, then let the air flow out slowly from your mouth or nose, as your hand goes back down.
- Completely exhale, and then repeat between five and ten times.
- If you experience light-headedness, stop the exercise for 30 seconds.

## *Muscle Relaxation*

Progressive muscle relaxation is an effective way to release tension and enhance the connection between body and mind. To do this, tense a body part and then let it relax. The contrast between exaggerated tightness and immediate looseness lets a warm feeling wash over your muscles.

How to Do It

- Sitting in a comfortable chair or lying down, close your eyes and place your hands at your sides or on your thighs. Breathe from your abdomen.
- For each body part, tense for 5 to 10 seconds, then immediately let go, relaxing for about 20 seconds. Allow yourself to feel your muscles loosening.
- Beginning from the bottom of your body, tighten the muscles of your feet by curling your toes, then release.

- Progressively work up your body, tightening then releasing your calves, thighs, buttocks, stomach, chest, shoulders, arms, and hands. For tensing your face muscles, try closing your eyes forcefully, raising your eyebrows high, opening your mouth wide, or smiling broadly.

## *Meditation*

The mind is fertile ground for negative thoughts, especially during stress. And when the mind worries, research shows, the ability to process information is disrupted—which is not good when you have to make important decisions every day.

Meditation offers a way to settle an anxious mind by focusing your attention on one thing—whether it's an object, your breath, or a word that you repeat, such as "one." During meditation, your thoughts will naturally wander—that's perfectly

---

### MEDITATION ON THE GO

Movement and meditation don't necessarily have to be separate. For some, the rhythm of a jog can bring calm. "Running is meditation on the move for me," says entrepreneur Mark Plaatjes. "It's a stress buster, and it makes me feel good. I can have a lot of things going on, and I pretty much work it out by the end of the run. I've come up with some of my best ideas while running."

Plaatjes, a world-class runner who won the marathon at the 1993 World Track & Field Championships, decided to turn his passion for the sport and his expertise as a physical therapist into successful business ventures. He co-founded Boulder Running Company in 1996 and also owns In Motion Rehabilitation, a physical therapy clinic.

Plaatjes uses the lessons he learned in competitive running to help him succeed in business. "With the marathon, you need to be very patient, and you need to make strategic moves at the right time," he says. In a retail business, he explains, patience also is a key when profits take time to show up as you pour money back into the business. And, he adds, thinking strategically is important as you consider when and where to expand, and what kinds of new lines you should add.

---

fine. Just gently refocus your attention on your "one thing," letting outside distractions simply pass through your mind without analysis. As Bourne explains in his workbook, "This process might be compared to watching leaves float by on the surface of a stream."

How to Do It

- Try meditating for just a few minutes at first. If you take a liking to it, you can eventually lengthen your sessions.
- Close your eyes if it makes you feel more relaxed.
- Don't judge how well you meditate or be concerned that you're not focusing well enough—that's not the point. Meditation offers a respite from the highly competitive and performance-driven parts of the rest of your day.
- A "meditation bowl" or "singing bowl" can provide a soothing sound to serve as an object of your focus (visit www.beinginharmony.com or www.freersacklershop.com/sounds.html).

---

### *Action* Items

➤ Keep track of how much sleep you get in the next five days—write this down on a notepad when you wake up in the morning.

➤ Take a minute to think about how much caffeine you drink during the day (including sodas), and whether you have trouble sleeping when you have caffeine late in the day.

➤ If you frequent a particular fast-food restaurant, visit its web site and take a glance at the nutrition breakdown. Are there some lower-fat, lower-calorie items you could choose?

---

> ### *Action* Items
>
> ➤ This week, try two yoga postures just before you go to bed.
>
> ➤ This week, take five minutes at your desk and do the breathing and muscle relaxation exercises.

## MOVEMENT AND AWARENESS GUIDELINES

Do these activities during breaks at work or during free time away from the office:

**Yoga Exercises**

| | |
|---|---|
| Cat Stretch | (repeat the sequence several times) |
| Twist | (one time each side) |
| The Warrior | (one time each side) |

**Deep Breathing**

Inhale and exhale from the belly up to 10 times or so

**Muscle Relaxation**

For each body part, tense for 5 to 10 seconds, then immediately let go, relaxing for about 20 seconds

**Meditation**

Practice for a few minutes at a time at first

# CHAPTER 12

# Healthy and Fit on the Go

*It was interesting being in Shanghai and Beijing. I left the hotel and went running for 45 minutes in one direction and then 45 minutes back. It was difficult because of the crowds of people, but then the bikers allowed me to run in their bike lanes. I didn't see a lot of runners in these major cities—most people bike—still, I felt camaraderie there.*

—STANLEY WUNDERLICH, CHAIRMAN AND CEO OF CONSULTING FOR STRATEGIC GROWTH 1 LTD.

## ONE-MINUTE SUMMARY

- You can reduce the effects of jet lag by adjusting your sleep schedule before you leave on your trip.
- Once you arrive, avoid scheduling meetings during the hours that correspond to your low energy points of the day back home; visit www.britishairways.com to determine your best times to seek out and avoid light to combat jet lag.
- Exercise also will help alleviate jet lag, so find out ahead of time if your hotel has an adequate fitness facility and check if the airport offers workout options.

> - Walking and running is a great way to see a city, get some local flavor, and stay on track with your fitness.
> - You can eat healthy meals at business lunches and dinners if you arm yourself with some simple strategies.

Nothing can derail your diet and fitness gains faster than a business trip. Faced with exhausting time-zone travel, fatty airline food, marathon meetings, and client dinners, your commitment to a healthy lifestyle is tested from the minute you board your plane. It's all too easy to slip out of your fitness mindset and into old habits. And the fatigue that can overcome you while traveling can hamper the focus you need to make your trip a success.

But it doesn't have to be this way. By making a few adjustments in your routine, you'll stay on track with your nutrition and fitness, and maintain the focus and energy you need when making important decisions for your business.

## AVOID THE JET-LAG DRAG

If you're flying over several time zones, you're at risk for jet lag, which results when your body's internal biological clock doesn't match up with local time. The effects can include insomnia, fatigue, lack of focus, irritability, and even mild depression—not the best ingredients for a prosperous trip. Jet lag may linger for more than a week when you fly across ten or more time zones. And ironically, the more experienced you are at business travel, the less likely you may be to take care of your sleep needs on the road, says Chris Idzikowski, Ph.D., a sleep expert who consults with British Airways on ways to ease jet-lag effects for passengers. "You're more likely to try to tough things out," he says.

Realize that you can be a smarter—and better rested—traveler by following some guidelines.

### *Adjust Ahead of Time*

Begin preparing your body for the time zone of your destination well before you leave for the airport. If possible, for several days before a trip west—which extends the hours in your day—make your bedtime and wake time one hour later each day. When traveling east—which shortens your day—do the opposite: make bedtime and wake time one hour earlier. Once you board the plane, reset your watch to reflect the time at your destination.

### *Realize Your Strengths and Weaknesses*

In general, traveling to the west tends to be easier on your body clock than traveling east. If you're a morning person, you may do better than a night person when traveling to the east; a night person may find it easier than a morning person when traveling west.

### *Get a Good Night's Sleep Before You Leave*

Take care of travel preparation well in advance so you don't shortchange your sleep before leaving. A study commissioned by Hilton Hotels & Resorts in cooperation with a former National Aronautics and Space Administration (NASA) fatigue expert looked at how the rigors of travel affected businesspeople, including their sleep, mood, and productivity. One of the biggest detriments to performance was—no surprise—sleep loss. But it turned out that the fewest hours of

---

## ORDER AHEAD

Call your airline or check online ahead of time to see if you can select a special meal for your flight—these may include servings that are vegetarian, gluten-free, low-sodium, or low-fat/low-cholesterol. Put in the request as soon as possible before your travel date. For a review of airline foods by actual passengers (including digital photos of meals), visit www.airlinemeals.net.

---

> *The best treatment for jet lag is water, water, and more water! Before long trips, I drink a quart of water before I get on the plane and as much as I can while in flight, ideally one large glass for every hour on the plane. Not only does it keep you from getting dehydrated, but because you have to make so many trips to the bathroom, it gives you an opportunity to move around and stretch.*
>
> —CLAIRE GRUPPO, FOUNDER AND CEO OF GRUPPO, LEVEY & CO.

sleep came the night before the trip, with participants averaging just five hours. "Essentially, travelers are at a decreased productivity level before they even walk out their door," commented Dr. Mark Rosekind, a former director of NASA's Fatigue Countermeasures Program. All told, the travelers had nearly eight hours of total sleep loss by the end of their trip.

### Bring Snacks and Sip Water

Airplane cabin air is very dry, with humidity ranging from 10 to 20 percent, so sip on water and avoid caffeinated and alcoholic drinks, which may dehydrate you. Pack healthy snacks such as fruit and nutrition bars in your carry-on. An inflight snack helps keep your energy level constant. Plus, having your own stash of fruit and nutrition bars once you get to your destination makes you less likely to succumb to hotel vending machines and other poor choices when the hunger pangs strike. Below are some nutrition bar options that provide fiber to fill you up but are relatively low in sugar so you avoid energy spikes and crashes. Just don't take along so many bars that you end up snacking *too* much—bring one for every day of travel, plus one for traveling out and one for the trip back if you have a long flight or layover.

- Odwalla Berries GoMega™ bar (110 calories; www.odwalla.com)
- Kashi Golean® Roll! Chocolate Peanut bar (190 calories; www.kashi.com)
- Organic Food Bar™ Original bar (300 calories; www.organicfoodbar.com)
- Larabar Apple Pie bar (190 calories; www.larabar.com)
- Clif® Nectar Cranberry, Apricot, and Almond Bar (170 calories, www.clifbar.com)
- Keribar™ (160 calories; www.keribars.com)

### Beware of Sleep Medications During Your Flight

Nonprescription sleep medicines can make you sleepy for a long time and make jet lag worse, warns the National Sleep Foundation. This means the effects could last well after you land. Talk to your doctor about a prescription sleep aid if you think it's necessary.

### Do Your Work Early in the Flight, Before You Sleep

Sleep helps lay down memory traces in the brain, Idzikowski says. "If you brief yourself for a meeting at the beginning of the flight prior to sleeping," he says, "the odds are you'll actually remember it better than if you cram the information at the end."

### Arrive in Time for a Good Night's Sleep

Try to schedule your trip for an arrival in the early evening so you can get to bed around 10 P.M. local time and enjoy a night of recuperative sleep. To foster good sleep, request a room away from elevators or ice machines, and bring something from home that will make you feel more comfortable—a photo or a light-reading book, for example. Schedule two wake-up phone calls in the event you sleep through one.

### Calculate When You Should Seek and Avoid Light

Idzikowski developed the "Jet Lag Advisor" for British Airways, which you can find on the company web site at www.britishairways.com/travel/sleep/public/ en_us. The tool is based on the concept that light is an important cue to manage our body clocks. You simply input answers to a few questions—what time you normally awaken in the morning, and the current time at your destination and at home—and the advisor gives you specific times you should either seek out or avoid light. By following the advice, you can achieve about three or four hours of time-zone adjustment in the first 24 hours, although results vary by individual. A "jet lag visor" can provide artificial light (Bio-Brite's is $250, at www.biobrite.com).

### Exercise

Exercise helps you adjust your body clock to a new time zone (see "Make Time for Exercise" later in the chapter for workout suggestions). In fact, in the Hilton

## SURVIVE THE RED-EYE

Getting any quality sleep on a red-eye flight is a tall order, but there are a couple of things you can do to help improve the chances you'll have at least some shuteye. Consider purchasing noise-reducing headphones (to minimize engine noise) and an eye cover to help encourage sleep. If possible, a seat that fully reclines is best (British Airways offers business-class seats that can lie flat). Not surprisingly, research shows that the quality of sleep worsens the more upright you are. A window seat may help by giving a place to rest your head.

You can also call the airline or check online to determine ahead of time the kind of airplane you're flying on. At www.seatguru.com, you can find detailed descriptions of good and bad seats listed by airlines and type of aircraft. (Exit rows may have more leg room but can be colder, for example). Lastly, avoid alcohol, which can disrupt sleep.

study mentioned earlier, business travelers who included exercise during their travels outperformed nonexercisers by 61 percent on tests of reaction and alertness.

### Schedule Meetings Strategically

The sleepiest time of day for our body clocks tends to be between 3 A.M. and 5 A.M. (and to a lesser extent between 3 P.M. and 5 P.M.). "It's sensible to have an awareness that that's your worst time for mental performance in your new time zone," says Idzikowski. Before the trip, figure out how these hours correspond with local time at your destination and, if possible, don't schedule important meetings during this period.

### Know Your Normal Wakeup Time

At your destination, you're likely to wake up at the hour corresponding with your wakeup time back home. If it's 3 A.M. and you can't fall back to sleep, that may be a time to do some more work, especially if it's a short trip. You could follow-up with a nap from 5 to 7 A.M. "By knowing when you're going to wake up," Idzikowski says, "you're not in a situation where you're stressed out because you can't control what's happening to you."

### Watch Out for Same-Time-Zone Trips

When you're traveling within the same time zone, fatigue still can be a problem although jet lag isn't. Daylight hours can be much shorter in northern cities than in southern cities in the winter, and so your sleep and mental outlook may still be affected.

### Don't Count on Melatonin

Melatonin has been a popular remedy for jet lag, but a 2006 study published in the *British Medical Journal* reviewed previous research and concluded that the evidence doesn't support melatonin as an effective treatment for jet lag. But if you're considering this supplement, talk with your physician first. It may help to cut down on the dose if melatonin doesn't work for you the first night, Idzikowski says. "You can swamp the effect by taking too high a dose, so it's worth backing off on it," he explains. If a reduced dose isn't effective the second night, he adds, give it up.

### Go Easy on Alcohol and Caffeine

In the Hilton business travel study, travelers boosted their alcohol consumption by 30 percent over what they drank at home. Caffeine consumption saw an increase

## DON'T LEAVE HOME WITHOUT IT

One of the most important things you need to pack doesn't take up any space—your fitness mindset. "Fitness is a part of me now, no matter where I am," says Robert Smith, president of Robert Smith & Associates Public Relations. "If I'm staying somewhere and they don't have a fitness room, I'll find a nearby park or somewhere to run."

## AVOID DEEP-VEIN THROMBOSIS

Deep-vein thrombosis, or DVT, happens when a clot forms in a leg vein and can be associated with limited mobility for extended periods. A person with DVT may experience leg pain, redness, or swelling, but with smaller clots, there may not be any symptoms. When a portion of the clot starts to travel to the lungs, serious injury or even death can result.

Some people may be more at risk because they already have a condition that affects circulation or normal blood clotting. Risk factors include an earlier case of DVT, heart disease, cancer, smoking, pregnancy, blood-clotting disorders, and advanced age. Even medications may be a risk factor for DVT—birth control pills and related hormones make some people a little more susceptible.

According to the Federal Aviation Administration, actions that may help include:

- Promoting blood flow by walking around or exercising your ankles and lower legs in your seat (see "Flexible Travel Arrangements" for some in-seat exercises you can perform)

- Wearing loose-fitting clothing to help prevent vein constriction

- Taking short naps rather than lengthy ones so you won't be inactive for too long

If you're at risk for DVT, talk to your doctor about what you can do. Special garments can decrease blood collecting in the legs, and medications may be used to thin the blood.

of 14 percent, with sodas the most popular caffeine source and coffee second. When you're away from your normal routine, it's easy to lose track of your consumption—but realize that these sources can worsen the effects of jet lag. Use caffeine wisely—it can promote alertness if you're fading (it generally takes effect in about 15 to 30 minutes), but depending on your sensitivity, it can cause sleep problems when taken too close to bedtime.

## MAKE TIME FOR EXERCISE

Exercise during your trip keeps you on pace with your fitness program as well as helps to alleviate the effects of jet lag, burns off stress, and gives you a sense of control over your environment. In the Hilton study, two-thirds of the business travelers surveyed said they exercised as a way to improve alertness, performance, and energy during their trip. Still, exercising on the road can be a challenge because of

---

## FLEXIBLE TRAVEL ARRANGEMENTS

To make the cramped quarters on your next flight a little easier to handle, and to help avoid deep-vein thrombosis, try these quick cabin stretches. These "stealth" exercises are so subtle your fellow passengers probably won't even catch on that you're exercising. For each, sit straight and tall in your seat and remember to keep breathing throughout. Take off your shoes or at least loosen the laces.

- *Foot flex.* Lift your heels off the floor and then lower them back down. Repeat this between 5 and 10 times. Then lift your toes off the floor and lower back down. Repeat this 5 to 10 times.

- *Foot rotation.* Lift your right foot a couple of inches and rotate your ankle a few times in a clockwise direction, and then reverse directions. Repeat with your left foot.

- *Overhead reach.* Interlock your fingers with palms facing out and slowly lift your arms straight overhead. Keep your shoulders relaxed and press your buttocks down while you stretch upward. Hold the position for 10 seconds, lower back down, and repeat twice. Do this stretch while walking around if overhead space in your seat is limited.

- *Torso twist.* Place your right arm across your chest. Grasp the right armrest with your left hand and gently twist your torso to the right, turning your head to the right and looking behind. Hold for 10 seconds, then repeat on the other side.

- *Shoulder shrug.* Hunch your shoulders up toward your ears and hold for 10 seconds, then let them relax and fall. Repeat twice.

---

> *I did a lot of traveling around Europe and Asia in my late 20s and 30s, and at that time, there weren't fitness clubs everywhere. I did the Jane Fonda aerobics routine in my hotel room, whatever time of day that it worked. And so I exercised even if all I had was a pair of running shoes, a pair of shorts, and a T-shirt.*
>
> —MARGARET MOORE, CEO OF
> WELLCOACHES CORPORATION

limited time and facilities. But there are some simple ways to make it more likely that you'll incorporate fitness away from home.

### Set a Schedule

When you travel, schedule your workouts just as you set appointments for meetings. Enter times in your personal digital assistant (PDA) or write them down in your appointment book before you leave. Morning workouts make the most sense because your end-of-the-day obligations can be uncertain when you're on the road. A morning workout also puts you in a healthy mindset for the rest of day, which will encourage you to make good food choices and get you feeling energized and confident.

### Pick a Healthy Hotel

You don't want to arrive at your lodgings to find that your workout option is an old conference room outfitted with a creaky exercise bike and a tattered floor mat. But if you don't plan ahead, that may be your luck. In a 2003 survey of 300 business travelers commissioned by Westin Hotels & Resorts, more than half said they had opted not to work out in a hotel fitness room because of its poor condition. Westin responded by teaming with Reebok to redesign its hotel fitness facilities to include weight machines, free weights, and high-quality cardio equipment with individual viewing screens for entertainment. Reebok also developed an in-room yoga- and Pilates-based workout you can do in bed.

Like Westin, other hotels seem to be cluing into the idea that business travelers want fitness options. In July 2006, Hilton Hotels Corporation announced plans to launch expanded fitness facilities at its North American full-service Hilton, Doubletree® and Embassy Suites Hotels®, as well as at its New York City-based The Waldorf=Astoria.

Visit www.fitforbusiness.com, a web site with an extensive database of business-friendly hotels that have either high-quality fitness facilities onsite or affiliations with a nearby gym. The web site, which does not accept payments from hotels and gyms for their listings, includes useful details such as the dumbbell weight range, the length of lap pools, and information on available business services. There are even international listings, including locations in Australia, Argentina, China, Italy, and the United Kingdom. The site is free, but a $50 annual fee gives you free or reduced-fee access to affiliated gyms, lower rates for personal training, time on racquet courts, and other services.

### Get a Passport

Another option for locating a gym in your destination city is the IHRSA Passport Program (IHRSA stands for the International Health, Racquet & Sportsclub Association). If you belong to a club in your hometown that participates in the program, then you're eligible for guest privileges at more than 3,000 other clubs worldwide (although you'll probably have to pay a guest fee). For more information, visit www.healthclubs.com.

Here are other helpful web sites for finding a workout on the road:

- *www.yogafinder.com.* A comprehensive listing of yoga classes in the United States and internationally, with links to local web sites.
- *www.indoorclimbing.com.* An international listing of climbing gyms and indoor rock climbing walls.
- *www.runtheplanet.com.* More than 4,000 descriptions, supplied by locals, of places to walk and run in more than 3,000 cities worldwide.
- *www.swimmersguide.com.* An international listing of full-size public swimming pools—with almost 16,000 pools in 156 countries.

### Work Out at the Airport

If you have a long layover or get to the airport early, why not get in some exercise? You can walk the concourse (travel in your walking or running shoes, or keep them in your carry-on) or even find a nearby gym that charges a one-time fee. Below is

> *I always try to stay in a hotel that has a gym or a fitness facility. That's one of the things I look for when I book hotels online. And because I travel so much, I have my favorites. If I go to New York, the Sheraton New York Hotel & Towers has a fabulous gym. The MGM Grand in Las Vegas is amazing, too.*
>
> —SUSAN SOLOVIC, CEO AND CHAIR OF SBTV.COM (SMALL BUSINESS TELEVISION)

a listing of airports with gyms in or attached to the terminal. For a comprehensive listing of more than 80 gyms in airports or within a short cab ride, visit www.airportgyms.com (most of the gyms charge a daily fee of around $5 to $15).

- *Boston.* At Boston's Logan International, a walk along a skybridge takes you to the Hilton, where there is a fitness room and pool.
- *Chicago.* The athletic club at the Hilton Chicago O'Hare Airport is accessible on foot from all airport terminals, and offers a lap pool and sauna.
- *Dallas/Fort Worth.* At the Dallas/Fort Worth International Airport, in Terminal D is the Grand Hyatt DFW, with its rooftop fitness center and pool.
- *Detroit.* The Westin located in the McNamara Terminal at the Detroit Metropolitan Airport features a WestinWorkout® powered by Reebok Gym and a pool, plus a running map designed by *Runner's World* magazine showing local three- and five-mile routes.
- *Las Vegas.* A 24 Hour Fitness club located in McCarran International Airport includes a sauna and a cardio area featuring big screen TVs.
- *Miami.* Miami International Airport Hotel, located inside Terminal E, has a health club that features a rooftop pool and a running track (the facilities are under renovation but are due to reopen in 2007).
- *Pittsburgh.* An enclosed walkway connects Pittsburgh International Airport to the Hyatt Regency and its health club, including a lap pool and sauna.

### Go for a Walk or Run

Walking and running are excellent exercise options when traveling because they require little extra in your luggage—just shoes and an outfit (take one workout outfit and rinse it out in the sink). Getting out on foot allows you to explore a city's hidden charms, scenery, and historical points. "When you travel, you're always in a hotel room or a conference center, and you don't really get out and see the city," says Gini Dietrich, president of Arment Dietrich. "Running allows you to do that."

Stephen Gatlin, CEO of Gatlin Educational Services, travels internationally for his business and has used his runs to explore the beachfronts in Cape Town, South Africa, and Dubai; Hyde Park in London; the boardwalk in Santa Monica, California; and parks in Brussels, Belgium and Amsterdam, the Netherlands. "It's a treat when the running habit allows you to experience some of the most lovely parts of cities," he says.

To find a local route near your hotel, ask the concierge or the front desk for a map and suggestions. When you're in unfamiliar territory, the safest bet is to pick an out-and-back route—it keeps you from getting lost, and it's easier to control the time you're out walking or running. Be cautious—trek with a colleague if possible and let someone know where you're going and how long you'll be gone. Be aware of your surroundings, avoid running or walking when it's dark, and use the side of the road where you face oncoming traffic. If you're not sure how safe an area may be, opt for the hotel's treadmill if one is available.

### Turn Your Room into a Gym

OK, suppose you don't have time to head outside or to a gym. No problem—do a scaled-down version of the resistance workout from Chapter 8 in your room. During his frequent business trips, Glenn Dietzel—CEO of the e-book consulting site www.awakentheauthorwithin.com and a start-up business advisor—does body weight exercises in his hotel room, keeping himself motivated by thinking about all the work he's put into his health and fitness. "It's the thought of losing some of what I've accomplished," he says, "that really keeps me focused."

Perform the following bodyweight exercises (from Chapter 8) once through, one after the other, with about 60 seconds' rest between exercises. Then repeat the circuit (so you'll complete a total of two sets per exercise). If you have some workout experience, you can reduce the rest to 30 seconds between exercises (this will keep your heart rate up and include a cardio component to the workout), and you can add a third set.

WORKOUT ON THE GO

|  | Repetitions | Sets |
|---|---|---|
| Two-leg floor bridge | 12 | 2 |
| Single-leg balance | 6–10 per leg | 2 |
| Push-up, standard or modified | 12–15 | 2 |
| Crunch | 15–20 | 2 |

Another good option is to pack lightweight resistance-training equipment:

- The AquaBells travel dumbbells fill with water ($60 for a pair; visit www.aquabells.com).
- JC Travel Bands are elastic exercise bands that fasten to a doorknob and come with exercise descriptions ($20, www.performbetter.com).
- Thera-Bands is another variety of elastic bands that are color-coded to signify different resistance levels and come with door anchors ($10 per band, www.thera-band.com).

## BE PREPARED FOR DINING OUT

If your business trip has you meeting with clients during lunch and dinner, plan ahead so you can arm yourself with some strategies that will keep you eating healthy while sealing your next deal. Don't worry about how a client may react to your healthy choices—public awareness of nutrition and obesity is prevalent these days, so it's perfectly acceptable to be open about wanting to eat a nutritious meal. And it's always possible that the client may find you to be an inspiration—making him even more loyal to your business. Keep these tips in mind, too, when ordering room service.

- Ask for a "small" or "medium" size for your entrée, any side dishes, and beverages. If entrees are still too big, make an appetizer your main dish or, if you know the client well enough, you may even propose splitting a meal.
- Order entrées that include veggies—for example, kebobs or a pasta dish with a tomato-based sauce. Instead of mashed potatoes or french fries, order a baked potato (without all the extras) or rice. For sandwiches, choose whole-wheat bread.
- Look for foods that have been baked, broiled, grilled, poached, roasted, or steamed—not sautéed or fried. Avoid foods with gravies or creamy sauces—or at least ask for sauce or gravy on the side, so that you have the option of controlling the amount you use.
- Order your salad dressing on the side. Dip your fork into the dressing and then into the salad. "This allows you to enjoy the smell and taste of the dressing without drenching every last piece of the salad, which can add 400 calories to a salad in dressing alone," nutritionist Kathy Wise says.

> ## CLIENT CONSIDERATIONS
>
> For business meals, if you choose the location, pick one you know has healthy options—both for yourself and your clients. "I have a client who is vegan," says SBTV.com's Susan Solovic. "I'm very cautious and aware of what kind of restaurants we go to, so there will be types of foods that she'll be able to eat."

- Always order water, even if you order another drink, because it will give you a no-calorie option on the table.
- Avoid meals made with mayonnaise, such as tuna or chicken salad, and order oil and vinegar instead of ranch or other creamy dressings.
- Ask your server if it's possible to have your meal made with low-fat cooking spray or with olive or canola oil, which are healthier monounsaturated fats. "There are a lot of different things that can go into a sauté pan," says Chad Luethje, executive chef at Red Mountain Spa, an active-oriented retreat in St. George, Utah, with a health-conscious clientele. "If you're lucky, it's going to be olive or canola oil. But more often than not, it's going to be clarified butter or something called Whirl®, which is a partially hydrogenated soybean oil with artificial butter flavoring."
- Beware the egg-white omelet. You may think this is a healthy choice, but cooks often use extra butter or oil to prevent sticking to the pan, Luethje says. You could be getting more fat and cholesterol than you would have just from the egg yolks. Ask your server if it's possible to cook using only olive oil. (For Chef Luethje's advice on cooking up healthy and flavor-packed meals, see Appendix C).
- The all-you-can-eat buffet is an invitation to gorge—avoid it and stick with a menu meal.
- If the menu is full of unhealthy foods, improvise. "Eat about half the meal," Wise says. "Try

> *I'm finding that the great news about restaurants today is they're extremely accommodating to people with healthy diets.*
>
> —DAN SANTY, FOUNDER OF SANTY ADVERTISING

spending more time talking to the client. And don't make a big deal of the fact that you're only eating part of it."

- Even if the menu offers healthy choices, give up the notion that you have to clean your plate—leave what you can't eat, or take leftovers in a doggie bag if you can get it to a refrigerator soon. Better yet, do a preemptive doggie bag—get one before you begin eating and stash half the meal away to reduce temptation.

---

### *Action* Items

➤ For your next business trip that crosses multiple time zones, plan several days in advance to shift your wake and sleep times (for several days before a trip west make your bedtime and wake time one hour later each day; when traveling east, do the opposite).

➤ Set specific times when you will exercise (preferably in the morning), just as you schedule business appointments during your trip

➤ Visit your hotel's web site to see if there is an adequate fitness facility on-site or close by; if necessary, visit www.fitforbusiness.com for other options.

➤ Pack fruit and nutrition bars for your flight and for your destination.

➤ Get in a workout, no matter how brief, every day of your trip.

---

# CHAPTER 13

# Healthy Considerations

> *When you're healthy, you feel good and you have more energy, which makes you more successful in your business. I think if you have that energy, it trickles down to your customers, vendors, and employees.*
>
> —JENNIFER MELTON, CO-FOUNDER OF CLOUD STAR NATURAL PET PRODUCTS

## ONE-MINUTE SUMMARY

- Common health conditions can often be controlled or avoided with smart lifestyle choices.
- Periodic screenings for particular conditions can detect health issues before symptoms show up, allowing for the most effective treatment.
- Losing weight and exercising can help decrease bad cholesterol and increase good cholesterol.
- The DASH (Dietary Approaches to Stop Hypertension) diet, in conjunction with reduced sodium intake, can help lower blood pressure.

> - Type 2 diabetes is dramatically on the rise—but a healthy diet, exercise, and modest weight loss can prevent or delay the onset of this disease.
> - Osteoporosis afflicts 55 percent of the population age 50 and older—but actions in your younger years can help in prevention.
> - Lifestyle changes could prevent half of all cancer cases in the United States, according to the Harvard Center for Cancer Prevention.

For a growing company, the health of the business is tied to the health of the entrepreneur. If you sneeze, the company is in danger of catching a cold. A disabling condition could put everything you've worked hard to build in jeopardy. As Richard Thompson, CEO and "Top Cat" of The Meow Mix Company, puts it: "You are your biggest asset. And if you don't take care of your biggest and best asset, you're not a very good entrepreneur."

Discuss your family's health history with your doctor—particular types of cancer, such as breast, colon, and prostate, tend to run in families, as do heart disease, stroke, high blood pressure, and diabetes. With this information, your physician will be better able to know if medications or lifestyle changes are important for prevention.

If you do have any health issues, staying on top of them will help minimize disruptions to your company. Of course, aside from your business, staying healthy allows you the vitality to enjoy all facets of your life.

In this chapter, you'll find a guide to some of the most common health conditions that could send your life and your business off track. Fortunately, they often can be avoided with smart lifestyle choices. Frequently these illnesses don't present any symptoms, so it's important to practice preventive health by getting regular screenings so you can head off problems and get effective treatment.

## CHOLESTEROL

Cholesterol is a waxy substance found in your bloodstream and cells. "It's not bad for you per se," says Steven Knope, M.D., author of *The Body/Mind Connection: Exploring the Undeniable Power of Strength* and a Tucson, Arizona-based physician whose patient base includes numerous entrepreneurs. "In fact, cholesterol is a needed component of all cells. When it becomes elevated, however, it can be a major risk factor for heart disease and stroke."

Cholesterol is produced in the liver, and the amount that's formed depends on the genetics passed on to you by your parents. To a lesser extent, cholesterol is controlled by what you consume in animal products such as eggs, butter, cheese, fish, meats, poultry, and whole milk. Foods with trans fat and saturated fat also stimulate cholesterol production.

Tiny packets known as lipoproteins carry cholesterol through the bloodstream. Low-density lipoproteins, or LDL, transport cholesterol out of the liver into other parts of the body. LDL cholesterol is called the "bad" cholesterol because if too much is circulating in the blood, deposits can build up and clog the arteries that lead to the heart and brain. The end result can be a heart attack or stroke.

On the other hand, high-density lipoproteins, or HDL, return cholesterol to the liver, and cholesterol is eventually eliminated from the body. Because HDL cholesterol helps clear out the arteries, it's called the "good" cholesterol.

---

### BEING THIN DOESN'T LET YOU OFF THE HOOK

While excess pounds can elevate cholesterol levels, a thin person should be just as aware of his numbers. "Most cholesterol elevations are due to genetics—what your parents gave you," says Steven Knope, M.D. Also, a person who doesn't put on weight easily may not be very conscious of the amount of saturated fat in his diet. As the American Heart Association says, "Nobody can 'eat anything they want' and stay heart healthy." So no matter how much you weigh, getting your cholesterol checked is a good idea.

---

An elevated cholesterol level doesn't cause any symptoms. But by checking your cholesterol numbers, you can take any necessary steps to bring them under control.

## Screening

Beginning at the age of 20, you should get screened every five years or more frequently if you have abnormal readings or any significant gains in weight. A full lipoprotein profile gives several important numbers:

- *Total cholesterol.* Less than 200 mg/dL (milligrams per deciliter) is considered desirable
- *LDL ("bad") cholesterol.* Less than 100 mg/dL is deemed optimal
- *HDL ("good") cholesterol.* Less than 40 mg/dL is considered low and a major heart disease risk factor; 60 mg/dL or higher can help reduce heart-disease risk
- *Triglycerides.* This is another type of fat found in blood that increases the risk of heart disease. Levels of 150–199 mg/dL are considered borderline high

## What You Can Do

Talk to your doctor about ways to control your cholesterol levels. Here are some important points to keep in mind.

- If you are overweight, losing excess pounds is a good place to start.
- Regular exercise can help decrease bad cholesterol and increase good cholesterol. However, the good cholesterol is primarily genetic. "To raise this level to a significant degree," Knope says, "you must do large volumes of aerobic exercise."
- As discussed in Chapter 6, saturated and trans fat increase blood levels of bad cholesterol. Trans fat also lowers good cholesterol. Recall that saturated fat is in animal foods such as cheese, whole milk, butter, ice cream, and fatty meats. You'll find trans fat in vegetable shortenings; some margarines; snack foods such as crackers and cookies; fried foods; doughnuts; baked goods; and other products containing partially hydrogenated oils.

## HEALTHY ALCOHOL?

"Alcohol is both a tonic and a poison," according to the Harvard School of Public Health. "The difference lies mostly in the dose." Alcohol in moderate amounts appears to benefit the heart and circulation, and also helps prevent gallstones and type 2 diabetes. A drink before eating can even help digestion.

Some research indicates that red wine has more advantages for the heart than hard liquor or beer, particularly if consumed with a meal, although one large study published in the *New England Journal of Medicine* in 2003 found heart benefits of moderate drinking across the board (beer, wine, or hard liquor). Red wine also contains antioxidants that may help inhibit certain cancers, according to the National Cancer Institute.

What's moderate? Limit daily drinks to one or two for men and one for women. One drink equals 5 ounces of wine, 12 ounces of beer, or 1½ ounces of hard liquor. Crossing over the line to heavier drinking can lead to liver problems, hypertension, stroke, and heart damage. For women, research shows that two or more daily drinks modestly raised breast cancer risk. (Daily folic acid intake of at least 600 micrograms may counter this risk). Alcohol, even in moderation, can cause sleep problems. For this reason, you shouldn't drink later in the evening.

Ultimately, the Harvard School of Public Health concludes that the benefits and risks of alcohol vary by individual, and that you should talk it over with your health-care provider. Harvard also notes that exercise and good nutrition can confer similar benefits. For more information, visit www.hsph.harvard.edu/nutritionsource/alcohol.html.

- Monounsaturated or polyunsaturated fats may decrease bad cholesterol and raise good cholesterol. Remember that olive and canola oils are sources of monounsaturated fats, while polyunsaturated fats are contained in nuts and fish, as well as corn, soybean, and sunflower oils.

- Soluble fiber may help decrease bad cholesterol, and good sources of fiber include oatmeal, oat bran, peas, brussels sprouts, carrots, beans, barley, rice bran, strawberries, citrus fruits, and apple pulp.

## HIGH BLOOD PRESSURE

High blood pressure, or hypertension, is a simple disease to diagnose and is easily manageable with lifestyle modifications or medications. As with high cholesterol there usually aren't any symptoms. Thirty percent of those who have the condition don't even realize it.

About one in three U.S. adults is afflicted with hypertension, which boosts the chances of heart disease and stroke, both top killers in the United States, and is also a major risk factor for congestive heart failure. High blood pressure causes your blood flow to exert greater force on the walls of the arteries, damaging them and eventually injuring organs. The condition also is linked with poorer cognitive performance.

### Screening

Blood pressure should be checked at regular doctor's office visits (along with body mass index). With a blood pressure reading, the top number (or systolic blood pressure) corresponds to the pressure on your arterial walls as your heart beats; the lower number (or diastolic blood pressure) indicates the pressure between heartbeats. These are the important numbers you need to know:

## PET DE-STRESSOR

A pet may do more than provide companionship—Fluffy and Fido may help moderate blood pressure. Research published in *Psychosomatic Medicine* compared people who owned dogs and cats with nonpet people. The finding: the pet owners enjoyed lower blood pressure, both while resting and under stress (performing math problems and dipping their hand in cold water).

## FINDING THE SILVER LINING

Optimism could possibly be strong medicine. In a study reported in the journal *Archives of General Psychiatry* in 2004, researchers found a link between positive outlook and decreased risk of death from heart disease and other causes in a group of men and women age 65 to 85 living in the Netherlands.

Optimism is also a boon to business, says Ray Smilor, Ph.D., the executive director of Beyster Institute at the Rady School of Management, University of California at San Diego, and former vice president of the Kauffman Center for Entrepreneurial Leadership at the Ewing Marion Kauffman Foundation. "Most people who build companies have a sense that things are going to get better," he says. "They view the glass half full, even when it's pretty much empty. They see the possibilities of things." The good news is that even if you're not naturally an optimist, it can be learned, says Smilor, who includes training sessions on developing a positive attitude in his seminars for entrepreneurs.

A good way to start is to watch how you label events. "I don't find many entrepreneurs who say, 'I failed,'" Smilor explains. Instead, for example, they'll say the timing just wasn't right for this particular technology. "When there's failure, they attribute it outside of themselves, and when there's success, they attribute it to themselves," Smilor says. "Labeling affects your perception. And if we label things differently, we can begin to see things in a different light and become a bit more optimistic about the challenges that we face."

- Normal blood pressure is systolic blood pressure of less than 120 mmHg and diastolic pressure of less than 80 mmHg.
- Prehypertension is a systolic reading of 120–139 mmHg *or* a diastolic measure of 80–89 mmHg (note that prehypertension is diagnosed by an elevation in one number or the other—it does not need to be both). Having prehypertension puts you at greater risk of developing high blood pressure.
- High blood pressure is 140 mmHg or greater for systolic pressure *or* 90 mmHg or greater for diastolic pressure (again, it can be one or the other).

- Beginning with a reading of 115/75, every increase of 20/10 doubles your chances of developing cardiovascular disease. Some physicians are becoming more aggressive in treating blood pressure and will begin treatment at 130/85.

### What You Can Do

If you have hypertension or prehypertension, talk to your doctor about your treatment options. Maintaining a proper weight, exercising, and healthy eating play important roles. The DASH (Dietary Approaches to Stop Hypertension) diet, in conjunction with lower sodium intake, is a nutrition program designed to lower blood pressure. "As opposed to a fad diet, such as the Atkins diet," Knope says, "the DASH diet is a legitimate diet that has been shown to reduce blood pressure to a level equivalent to drug monotherapy (one drug) in just two weeks." For more information, visit www.nhlbi.nih.gov/health/public/heart/hbp/dash.

Also, stress may contribute to hypertension—cortisol and adrenaline released during stressful situations narrow blood vessels and increase heart rate. To bring calm to your day, practice the awareness techniques described in Chapter 11.

### DIABETES

Diabetes is a disease that disrupts the body's insulin regulation. The most prevalent form of the condition is type 2 diabetes, accounting for up to 90 percent of

### MALE PROBLEMS

Men die an average of 5.4 years sooner than do women, according to The Men's Health Network, a group promoting awareness of male health. Men also die at higher rates than women from the ten leading causes of death, including diabetes, suicide, heart disease, and cancer. And yet, men are much less likely than women to see a doctor for checkups. Unfortunately, one possible reason is that men may view visiting a physician as a sign of weakness.

## HOLD THE FRIES

A study published in 2006 in the *American Journal of Clinical Nutrition* found a link between type 2 diabetes and eating potatoes, especially when in the form of french fries. One reason may be that potatoes are high on the glycemic index (GI), which means they trigger a quick spike in blood sugar. In the long run, this can disrupt the body's insulin regulation. Substituting whole grains—which offer a lower GI—for potatoes and white-flour foods may help reduce diabetes risk.

the cases of diabetes (the other types are type 1 diabetes, which typically strikes young adults and children, and gestational diabetes, which afflicts between 2 and 5 percent of women during pregnancy). Certain ethnic groups are at greater risk for diabetes, including African Americans, Asian Americans, and Hispanic Americans.

Insulin, a hormone produced by the pancreas, helps shuttle glucose (or blood sugar) from the food we consume into cells throughout the body, where the glucose is converted into energy. Early on in type 2 diabetes, the body is able to make enough insulin for its needs, but is unable to make effective use of insulin. This is what is called "insulin resistance." Over time, the pancreas wears out, insulin levels fall, and glucose backs up in the blood—as a result, patients must take oral medications or insulin through a syringe.

Diabetes is diagnosed when at least two fasting glucose readings are measured at 126 mg/dL or above. Prediabetes occurs when levels of blood glucose are above normal but are not high enough to be considered diabetic. Prediabetes puts you at greater risk for type 2 diabetes, stroke, and heart disease.

Diabetes can seriously harm vital body parts—the kidneys, heart, blood vessels, nerves, eyes, feet, legs, gums, and teeth—and result in blindness and lower-limb amputations. It is also a major cause of erectile dysfunction. Risk factors for the disease include being overweight or obese, keeping a sedentary lifestyle, having gestational diabetes, having a baby that weighs more than nine pounds at birth, and having a family history of diabetes. As more and more people have become overweight and obese in the United States, there's been an increase in type 2 diabetes—now about 20.8 million people are affected, according to a statement issued in 2006 from the National Institutes of Health.

## *Screening*

In general, you should be tested for diabetes if you are 45 years of age or older, and then every three years. But people at high risk should be checked before age 45—talk to your doctor about your own situation. Type 2 diabetes is a disease that may not cause any symptoms, but you may notice at least one of these signs, according to the U.S. Department of Health and Human Services:

- Being very hungry or thirsty
- Frequent urination (particularly at night)
- Feeling very tired
- Weight loss without trying
- Sores that heal slowly
- Tingling or numbness in the hands or feet
- A sudden change in vision

## BACK ON TRACK

The early stage of starting up SBTV.com, a television network on the internet aimed at small businesses, took a toll on entrepreneur Susan Solovic. "In the first year, I really started seeing my health deteriorate because I wasn't paying attention to what I knew I needed to do," she says. Experiencing debilitating back pain, she decided to take charge of her health. "I just said: 'You know, this is ridiculous. This is my body, I'm in control of it, and I'm just not going to let this happen. From this day forward my health, my body, is a priority. That's just the way it's going to be.'"

Solovic began working out and watching her nutrition, and now she's seeing the payoff. Although her back pain is not completely gone, exercise helps to minimize its effect, she says. "I have more energy, my mood is better, I'm happier," she adds. "It's amazing. I just feel so much better."

- More infections than usual (including vaginal yeast and bladder infections in women)
- Stomach pain, vomiting, or nausea

### What You Can Do

Because the biggest risk factors for developing type 2 diabetes are excess weight and a sedentary lifestyle, start there. "If you are overweight, you should try to lose weight," says Knope. "Even losing 10 to 15 pounds is enough to allow many patients to come off of their medications." Even if you're unable to lose weight, he adds, exercising moderately–such as walking two to four times per week for 30 minutes—can reduce your risk of developing diabetes by 30 percent.

## OSTEOPOROSIS

Osteoporosis involves bone loss that can lead to fractures. According to the National Osteoporosis Foundation (NOF), about 10 million people in the United States have the disease, while nearly 34 million more suffer from low bone mass, putting them at greater risk for developing osteoporosis. All told, 55 percent of the population age 50 and older is affected, reports NOF. And although the disease typically is associated with women, about 2 million of those afflicted are men.

The bone loss that comes with osteoporosis doesn't present symptoms—that is, until a person suffers a fracture. And chances are good this will happen. Fifty percent of women and 25 percent of men older than age 50 will endure a fracture that is osteoporosis-related in their remaining lifetime, according to NOF. On average, almost a quarter of those people who fracture a hip when age 50 and older die in the following year. Six months postfracture, only 15 percent can walk unassisted.

To understand what causes osteoporosis, it's helpful to understand that your bones are in a constant

> *I started doing yoga because my mother has very bad osteoporosis, and so I was concerned about my risk for developing the disease. Through yoga, I wanted to build upper body strength.*
>
> —NANCY LeClaire, WHO OPERATES FINANCIAL PLANNING EDUCATIONAL SOLUTIONS, A BUSINESS THAT TRAINS FINANCIAL PLANNERS

## POWERFUL MEDICINE

Overwhelmingly, the medical literature supports the idea that the most important things you can do to maintain your health are exercising regularly and eating well, says Steven Knope, M.D. "If you do only those things, your chances of remaining healthy increase dramatically," Knope says. "If you do one thing, exercise regularly."

state of change. Throughout life, their structure is continually broken down and reconstructed. If you're sufficiently active and consume enough calcium, your body builds more bone than is lost until age 30 or so. Beyond this age, the breakdown process overtakes the building process.

Bone loss with age has roots in multiple factors, including heredity, being physically inactive, and reduced hormone levels—estrogen for women and testosterone for men. In fact, in the early years following menopause, women can suffer a bone-mass loss of as much as 20 percent.

### Screening

Talk with your doctor about your particular risk for osteoporosis. A bone-density test is painless and can find osteoporosis before you suffer a fracture. A physician will typically recommend a screening for women entering menopause. Also, any woman who is 65 or older should get one (younger postmenopausal women should, too, if they have a risk factor such as family history of osteoporosis). Men who have any indication of low testosterone (erectile dysfunction or loss of libido) should have a screening for testosterone level. If the reading is low, they should have a bone-density study.

### What You Can Do

Maximizing bone growth up to the age of 30 is important for preventing osteoporosis later in life. In adulthood, your aim should be to limit bone loss, and some lifestyle strategies can help, including:

REGULAR EXERCISE. Weight-bearing activities—such as walking, jogging, hiking, resistance training (for example, the exercises described in Chapter 8), and racquet sports—stress the bones, and they respond by maintaining or possibly even adding density. Also, resistance training confers muscle strength that can help decrease the chances of falling.

CALCIUM INTAKE. The body uses calcium to build bones and teeth, and for blood clotting, regulating heart rhythm, and conducting nerve impulses. The recommended daily intake is 1,000 mg for people age 19 through 50, and 1,200 to 1,500 mg for those 51 or older. Women 19 and older who are pregnant or lactating are advised to get 1,000 mg per day. (According to the Harvard School of Public Health's web site at www.hsph.harvard.edu, the safest and healthiest level of calcium intake is still unclear. Talk to your doctor about what is best for your situation.)

Milk and dairy products are sources of calcium, but it's also present in other foods, such as dark green leafy vegetables (for example, broccoli, collard greens,

## PRIORITIZING

Dan Santy, who heads Santy Advertising, has a fitness routine that includes weight training three days a week, indoor cycling, and hiking Camelback Mountain near his home in Phoenix, Arizona. His pursuits give him an "incredible lift mentally and physically," he says, sustaining his energy for working long hours.

Santy watches his diet closely, eating fruits and vegetables, and favoring lean protein sources such as turkey and chicken to help build muscle. His advice for staying fit and healthy? "Make it an important part of your day," he says. "I'm a morning guy, so my routine is in the morning before work. I set my schedule, and I say it's a priority. It's as important as anything that I do for my clients or my company."

Success in business parallels incorporating a healthy lifestyle, he adds. "Do a few things and do them well," he says. "Find out what it is you like. If it's Spinning®, then go spin. If you're a runner, go run. Determine what works for you—what's at your core—and focus on it. That focus is important for success in both business and exercise."

## CAFFEINE AND CALCIUM

Drinking four or more cups of coffee each day may raise the chances of a bone fracture. That's because caffeine fosters calcium loss in urine.

and kale), and in legumes. Calcium supplements and calcium-fortified orange juice, breads, and cereals provide still more sources.

VITAMIN D. Vitamin D is important for the absorption of calcium. It's present in foods such as milk, egg yolks, and saltwater fish. The skin also makes vitamin D when exposed to sunlight—although the winter sunshine in Northern regions (north of Philadelphia and San Francisco) is too weak for vitamin D production. Many multivitamins and some calcium supplements provide vitamin D. A recommended intake is 400 to 800 international units (IU) per day, and the National Osteoporosis Foundation advises not exceeding 800 IU per day unless prescribed because high amounts could be harmful.

VITAMIN K. This vitamin is important in regulating calcium and is present in green leafy veggies. The daily recommended amount for men is 120 micrograms and for women is 90 micrograms. Eating at least one daily serving of broccoli, collard greens, brussels sprouts, kale, or dark green lettuce should do the trick.

## CANCER

Cancer involves uncontrolled growth of cells in a particular area of the body. In the United States, the disease is the second leading killer—but survival rates are improving with earlier diagnosis and new and improved treatments.

### Screening

Regular cancer screenings are important cancer-prevention tools. According to the American Cancer Society (ACS), the five-year rate of survival for patients with cancers of the colon, rectum, breast, cervix, testes, prostate, skin, and oral cavity is about 82 percent (this excludes those who die from other causes). The society estimates that if every American followed recommendations for early detection testing, the five-year rate of survival for these cancers would be about 95 percent.

When having periodic health checkups, in addition to the specific tests given below, the ACS advises that, depending on age, a cancer-related exam might include checks for cancers of the oral cavity, thyroid, skin, testes, lymph nodes, and ovaries. The following are general guidelines—some physicians may advise earlier screenings, especially if you have certain risk factors, so talk with your doctor about what's best for you.

- *Clinical breast exam (CBE) and mammography.* Have a CBE every three years up to age 40, then have one on a yearly basis along with a mammogram.
- *Pap test.* Have one each year from age 20 to 30; from age 30 on, have a test every one to three years, depending on the individual recommendations you get from your doctor. (In June 2006, the U.S. Food and Drug Administration approved a vaccine that is effective against a majority of cervical cancers, for use in females 9 to 26 years old—although regular pap tests are still required.)
- *Colon/rectal screening.* Different testing options exist; a colonoscopy is the most effective and checks the entire colon. For his average-risk patients, Knope recommends a colonoscopy at the age of 50. If there aren't any polyps or abnormalities seen, this is repeated in 10 years. Between ages 55 and 60, patients complete stool cards for occult blood every year. If abnormalities are found, a colonoscopy is done more frequently.
- *Prostate exam.* For average-risk patients, Knope advises screening beginning after the age of 40 with a digital prostate exam. Depending on the physician,

## TOMATO POWER

A substance found in tomatoes called lycopene, which gives tomatoes their red color, may help protect against prostate cancer (cooked tomato products may be the most beneficial).

PSA (prostate-specific antigen) blood testing may be started at age 50 or at age 40 to 45 for African-American men or men with a family history of prostate cancer.

### What You Can Do

Lifestyle factors have a big effect on cancer risk. In fact, according to the Harvard Center for Cancer Prevention, half of all cancer cases in the United States could be prevented by lifestyle changes—avoiding weight gain and tobacco, eating well, reducing alcohol consumption, and boosting physical activity. "Cancers that are particularly responsive to exercise prevention include breast cancer, colon cancer, and ovarian cancer—all of which are reduced by about 30 percent with regular exercise," Knope says.

Higher intake of veggies and fruits is linked with a reduced risk of various cancers, according to the World Health Organization's International Agency for Research on Cancer. And not getting adequate amounts of vitamins raises the chances of chronic disease, including cancer, as well as osteoporosis and cardiovascular disease. Unfortunately, according to the Harvard School of Public Health, many people don't get enough vitamins B-6, B-12, D, and E, or enough folic acid, which may help decrease the risks of breast cancer and colon cancer. Although a multivitamin/mineral supplement isn't a substitute for a healthy diet, it can help ensure that you're meeting your daily needs in these and other nutrients.

---

### *Action* Items

➣ Review the list of important screenings to determine if you've had any recently.

➣ If you're due for any of the screenings, schedule an appointment with your doctor in the next several weeks, and talk about which checkups he or she recommends.

---

## SCREENINGS SUMMARY

Screenings can detect health problems even before symptoms arise, allowing the most effective treatment:

___ *Cholesterol check.* Beginning at the age of 20, every five years, or more often if levels are abnormal or there is any significant gain in weight.

___ *Blood pressure and body mass index.* During each regular visit to the doctor's office.

___ *Blood-glucose (sugar) test.* Every three years beginning at the age of 45 (but sooner if at high risk).

___ *Bone-density test for osteoporosis.* For women entering menopause, women 65 or older, and younger postmenopausal women if they have a risk factor; also, men with low testosterone level.

___ *Clinical breast exam (CBE) and mammography.* CBE every three years up to age 40, then annually along with a mammogram.

___ *Pap test.* Each year from age 20 to 30; from age 30 on, test every one to three years depending on physician recommendations.

___ *Colon/rectal screening.* Colonoscopy at the age of 50. If there are no polyps or abnormalities, repeat in 10 years. Between ages 55 and 60, annually complete stool cards for occult blood. If abnormalities exist, a colonoscopy is performed more frequently.

___ *Prostate exam.* Digital prostate exam starting after the age of 40. Possibly a PSA test beginning at age 50, or at age 40 to 45 for African-American men or men with prostate cancer in their family history.

You may need other screenings, or again you may require testing when younger, depending on your medical history, ethnicity, and the medical history of your family (for example, if a close relative was diagnosed with colorectal cancer before age 60). Also, you may want to discuss with your doctor the possibility of a cardiovascular stress test.

For more information, visit:

- *www.everydaychoices.org.* A joint web site of the American Cancer Society, the American Diabetes Association, and the American Heart Association.

- *www.ahrq.gov/ppip/healthywom.htm, www.ahrq.gov/ppip/healthymen.htm, www.womenshealth.gov/Tools.* U.S. Department of Health and Human Services web sites with information on recommended health screenings for men and women.

# CHAPTER 14

# Staying Motivated

*A lot of guys who do the Ironman CEO Challenge are really exceptional athletes—former cyclists or swimmers or runners. But then there are other people like me, more average Joes in triathlon, who just decide that it would be really cool to try an Ironman®. So they do it.*

—MIKE NAGEL, VICE PRESIDENT OF SALES AND MARKETING FOR INCISIVE SURGICAL AND CO-FOUNDER OF VASCULAR SOLUTIONS INC.

## ONE-MINUTE SUMMARY

- Now that you've started implementing your new healthy habits, it's important to maintain your motivation by keeping things fresh.
- Signing up for an event, such as a 5K run, bike tour, or triathlon gives you a clear fitness goal and channels your entrepreneurial self-discipline and competitiveness.
- Taking an active vacation allows you to put your fitness into action and helps prevent burnout.

> ⊛ Joining a gym gives you access to specialized equipment and classes, as well as a supportive environment.
>
> ⊛ Working with an experienced trainer or wellness coach can take your fitness to another level and make you accountable to another person— and more likely to stick with your program.

With exercise and good nutrition becoming more and more a part of your life, you're entering the maintenance stage of change that we looked at in Chapter 5. It's in this stage that you solidify your healthy behaviors so that they last a lifetime.

It's also in this stage that you risk complacency and boredom. Even though you've made it this far, a relapse to old habits is a possibility—and you need to make sure that you maintain your motivation, especially in the early going when you're still testing the waters of your new lifestyle. In short, if you don't keep your program fun and interesting, it's easy to stray off course.

Keeping things fresh is pretty simple if you plan ahead. By incorporating some key lifestyle strategies, you'll stoke the fire of your motivation to keep it burning in the days, months, and years ahead.

## DO AN EVENT

A surefire way to stay motivated is to sign up for an organized event, such as a 5K or 10K run (3.1 and 6.2 miles, respectively), a bicycle tour, or a triathlon. By sending in an entry fee two to three months in advance, you give yourself a definite goal and a built-in time line to get it done. If you have the typical entrepreneurial drive, competitiveness, and self-discipline, participating in an athletic event is a great way to channel those traits into something that makes you healthier.

In reality, organized rides, runs, and triathlons are more celebrations of the human spirit than they are races. Spectators often line the course to cheer you on, while after the race exhausted but exhilarated athletes share war stories of their experiences. The rush of adrenaline when you cross the finish line combined with the genuine sense of camaraderie with the other competitors makes for a day you'll always remember.

Check these resources to find local bike rides, triathlons, and runs:

- Web sites such as www.active.com or www.competitor.com, where you can sign up online
- Regional sports-specific magazines, often found in health clubs
- Neighborhood bike or running stores

Doug MacLean, co-founder of Talking Rain, whose products include sparkling water and vitamin-enhanced water, ran cross-country and track in high school but didn't get back to his competitive ways until entering running events in his late 30s. Since then, he's embraced the sport fully. "If I go on vacation, I look for races," he says. "If I travel to Europe, I look for races. It just becomes part of your life."

Stephen Gatlin, CEO of Gatlin Educational Services, started by signing up for 5Ks and now likes to run half-marathons (13.1 miles). "Having an event coming up always causes me to use the same project management skills I use in business to

## TEAMING UP

If you can make the time, joining a sports league is another way to invigorate your routine and satisfy your competitive ambitions. Sports such as basketball, volleyball, and hockey have scheduled practices and games, plus a group of people relying on your ability to stay fit. For Dan O'Shea, who quit smoking 15 years ago and now has a regular fitness routine, playing in a competitive inline-skating hockey league helps keep him in the best shape of his life. "It's a release," says O'Shea, who with his wife Suzy Jurist co-owns SJI Associates, an advertising and design firm. "For the hour and a half that I'm playing, I concentrate on nothing but hockey—and it makes me feel young." To find leagues in your area, check with your city's recreation department.

> *I think it's critical to find a workout partner who has similar goals, or maybe somebody who's just slightly ahead of you, to provide motivation. I don't know too many people in the world who are disciplined enough if they don't have a partner, especially in the early going. If you know your buddy is waiting for you and you've agreed to meet at 5:30 in the morning, you're going to get up and go do it. If the only thing that's waiting for you is a cold bike or a cold windy day, it's too easy to skip it.*
>
> —DAN SANTY, FOUNDER OF SANTY ADVERTISING

make sure I'm ready," he says. "For example, if there is a 10K in a month, I know I need to run an hour a couple of times a week if I am going to be prepared."

Keep in mind that cycling events, 10Ks, marathons, and even Ironman® triathlons are not reserved for top athletes—in fact these sports are appealing in large part because all levels of ability are welcome. Here democracy is applied to sport—everyone showing up at the starting line is created equal because everyone is testing his or her own unique limits.

Entrepreneur Mike Nagel took up doing triathlons about five years ago and has been hooked ever since. By starting with shorter races, Nagel says he was able to gradually work up his modest athletic ability to compete in Ironman® triathlons—a 2.4-mile swim, 112-mile bike ride, and 26.2-mile marathon done one after the other. "I decided a few years ago, if I'm going to do it, do it big," says Nagel, who participates in the CEO Ironman Challenge (www.ceochallenges.com).

Whether you ever decide to take things as far as Nagel, realize that running just a few days a week could prepare you for a 10K in a few months time. One of the best ways to train for an event is to find a training group. This provides a supportive atmosphere with like-minded people and work-out partners, a fun social environment, and often a knowledgeable coach to help guide you to your goal. This also makes your training more efficient by reducing your risk of injury—making it less likely that you'll be wasting your time.

Check with local running and biking shops to see if they know of any training groups. Often, informal and structured athletic groups get together to train, with room for any level of ability. For swimming, contact your local college or public lap pools for classes and organized workouts.

The following programs are formalized national programs offering support in training for running, biking, and/or triathalon events:

- *Jeff Galloway's Training Programs.* The long-time running coach and *Runner's World* columnist advocates a run-walk program that can have you doing a marathon in six months if currently you can run or walk three miles. Training groups are offered in more than 45 cities (www.jeffgalloway.com).
- *Team in Training.* Operated through The Leukemia & Lymphoma Society, this program provides training for a marathon, half-marathon, century bike ride (100 miles), or an Olympic-distance triathlon (approximately 1-mile swim, 25-mile bike, and 6.2-mile run). You also receive free travel, hotel, and entry to the race, while you're expected to raise funds for the society (www.teamintraining.org).
- *National AIDS Marathon Training Program.* Training programs for half-marathons and marathons are currently offered in the Los Angeles, San Francisco, Chicago, and Washington, DC areas. You raise funds for AIDS services, and the program provides free travel, accommodations, and race entry (www.aidsmarathon.com).

## TAKE AN ACTIVE VACATION

Taking a break from your business—even for just a long weekend—can help you avoid burnout and recharge your enthusiasm. But, instead of the same-old sitting-on-the-beach getaway, put your fitness to good use with a more active vacation. Seeing a destination from the seat of a mountain bike or

*On a trip to Montana a couple of summers ago, I signed up, on the spur of the moment, for a day of "rock climbing for beginners." I had never even been on a climbing wall in the gym. The other "beginners" were all in their 20s, extremely fit, and strong. With a little instruction, all the appropriate equipment, and the careful watch of our guide, I was able to scale 1,500 feet of sheer rock, get to the top first, and look out over the most glorious scenery imaginable! It was thrilling, at 51, to be able to enjoy that experience.*

—CLAIRE GRUPPO, FOUNDER AND CEO OF GRUPPO, LEVEY & CO.

## THE ROAD TO SUCCESS

Entrepreneur Stacy Madison took on a big challenge when she signed up for the New York-to-Boston AIDS Ride—a 350-mile bicycling event. Madison came up with the idea after talking to a friend who had done the ride with her husband. "They weren't avid cyclists, and they didn't work out all the time," she remembers. "At the time I was probably in the best shape of my life, so I thought, 'Why couldn't I do something like this?'"

In training for the ride, she picked up tips and strategies by participating in periodic organized training rides on weekends. "My goal wasn't to break any records," says Madison, who launched Stacy's Pita Chip Company with Mark Andrus in 1997. "My goal was simply to ride from New York to Boston and not get off my bike when I had to go uphill." The four-day ride, she says, "was awesome. It was an experience of a lifetime."

To find entrepreneurial success, Madison advises, take advantage of available resources, such as classes and community services offered to new businesses. "There are lots of services specifically targeted to women who are starting a business," she says. "And don't be afraid to ask for help and to ask questions. The worst that can happen is somebody says no, and then you pick up the phone and ask somebody else."

A former social worker, Madison says you don't necessarily need to have a background in the specific business area you're entering. "Think of all of your own life experiences," she says, "and pull what you can from that to be successful."

from the perspective of a local hiking trail brings you closer to the real charm of a location, with the satisfaction of knowing that you're doing it under your own power.

Adventure vacations run the gamut from back-country hiking and camping to kayaking and whitewater rafting to more leisurely bike rides with overnight stays in top hotels. Some travel companies offer expert guides, while others help outfit you with the proper gear and then let you explore on your own. And while some trips require a pretty good level of fitness, others are accommodating to those just getting into shape. Whatever your preference, there's most likely an outfitter that will be more than willing to meet your needs.

America Outdoors (www.americaoutdoors.org) is a travel trade association of more than 600 outfitters that provide trips in the United States and around the world. The association operates the web site www.adventurevacation.com, where you can search for trips by state or region, and by activity type.

Multiday trips can book up well in advance, so for longer trips plan at least six months ahead. When you're looking into a particular vacation, questions for the tour operator include:

- How long has the company been in business?
- How long has the company covered this particular adventure trip and destination?
- How experienced is the guide, and is he or she CPR certified?
- For camping trips, will the guide be responsible for setting up camp and cooking?
- What level of fitness will I need?
- What type of equipment and gear and clothing will I need to bring?
- Will families/children be in the group?
- What are the names and contact information of a few people who have gone on this particular trip?
- Does the quoted price include everything? (A tip for your guide probably won't be included.)
- What kind of cancellation policy do you have?

Some of the established tour operators are:

- *REI Adventures.* With nearly two decades of adventure travel experience, REI guides trips all over the world, and adventures include walking, kayaking, rafting, and cycling. The group size is usually fewer than 16 people, and trips are rated from easy to vigorous (www.rei.com/adventures).
- *Gorp Travel.* Gorp offers an online resource for finding adventure vacations, and you can search for trips by region and activity, including biking, hiking,

climbing, paddling, horseback riding, and snow sports (www.gorp travel.com).

- *Sierra Club.* Founded more than a century ago, the club now organizes more than 350 worldwide adventures, including backpacking, biking, and canoe trips, with small groups led by volunteer guides (www.sierraclub.org).
- *Backroads.* Another longtime outfitter, Backroads offers 230 trips covering 90 destinations on six continents. You'll have options for walking, hiking, biking, and multisport trips. Depending on the package, accommodations range from camping to "Premiere Inns," where you stay overnight at five-star hotels and dine on fine cuisine (www.backroads.com).

## JOIN A GYM

While exercising at home or in your office is effective, there are certain perks to joining a gym. At many facilities you have access to a wide array of fitness equipment; specialized group classes, such as kickboxing and yoga; and personal trainers who can evaluate your current fitness level and goals and design a training program tailored to your needs. You meet other people with similar objectives, providing more support for your efforts to stay on track. And when you're paying good money for something, you're more likely to use it.

"In the morning, I'll go to the gym for about a half-hour to 45 minutes," says Dominic Rubino, a business coach who owns the Fulcrum Agency, a consulting agency in Vancouver, British Columbia, and who is a member of the Young Entrepreneurs Association. "I hop on the StairMaster or elliptical trainer, get a good sweat going, and start thinking about the day." After work, Rubino heads to the gym for a kickboxing and ground-grappling class. "I've been in martial arts for a good portion of my life, and it's just a really good workout," he says. "As an entrepreneur, you spend the whole day telling other people what to do. But then in a martial arts class, you have no choice—when the sensei [teacher] tells you to do something, you do it."

Sometimes it takes a little creativity to squeeze in time for the health club. Investment banker Claire Gruppo takes advantage of the flexibility of being an entrepreneur and gets in a gym workout when the time is right—even if that

## TEN (MORE!) WAYS TO STAY MOTIVATED

1. Watch *Rocky* (or another inspiring guy/gal-overcomes-the-odds movie).

2. Listen to your favorite upbeat music ten minutes before you exercise.

3. Promise yourself your favorite dessert tonight if you run this morning (just don't make this one a daily habit!).

4. Tell your friends and family about your new exercise and diet—it makes you more accountable.

5. Take a minute to visualize yourself *after* your workout—relaxed, energized, and enjoying the satisfaction of accomplishing your goals.

6. Make friends with or date someone who exercises.

7. Oftentimes, just getting out the door and making it one block is the most difficult part of aerobic exercise. Tell yourself you'll just walk to the end of the block and see how you feel—usually once you get to the end of the block you feel like going a little farther. But even if you don't, that's fine. At least you did something!

8. Give $100 to a friend and tell her it's hers to keep if you don't walk/run three days a week for the next month.

9. Pick a new route to walk or run, instead of the same old path you've gotten used to. On the weekend, drive to a neighborhood you've wanted to see and go exploring on foot.

10. Keep a log of your workouts—even just a few days worth of jogs or walks starts to look impressive when you see it in writing.

means it's at 4:30 in the afternoon. "In a highly demanding job, where people are after you all the time, the second it's quiet, you have to just leave and you go to the gym," she says.

**TIME SAVER TIP**

Join a gym that's near work or on the way—this won't just save time, it'll make it more likely you'll go. "I have to pass the gym on my way home," says Mark Andrus, co-founder of Stacy's Pita Chip Company. "So there's really no excuse to skip my workout."

Terri Alpert, who runs Uno Alla Volta LLC, rarely schedules appointments with vendors or employees before 11 A.M., so she always has time to get in a morning workout. "Occasionally there's something really important I have to make the exception for," she says. "But I try to make it a huge exception. Because otherwise it's too easy to fall back into the pattern that I used to have, which was 'I'll go to the gym if there's time.'"

Choose your facility carefully—there are more than 26,000 clubs nationwide, and the quality can differ. Monthly dues are typically $55, according to the International Health, Racquet, and Sportsclub Association, but fees will vary by location and by the extent of services and facilities.

Remember to inquire about the credentials of the staff. Questions to ask include:

- Are staff members qualified in CPR, automated external defibrillators, and first aid?
- If you have a special medical condition such as high blood pressure, does the club have a program to address this?
- Will you be given a pre-exercise health screening?
- Are complimentary personal training sessions available with a new membership?
- Does the club offer a trial membership? (It may take a couple of weeks of going to the gym at different times to see if the atmosphere is right for you.)

## GET PERSONAL

Working with a good personal trainer can be an effective way to launch your fitness program or motivate you if you've hit a bump in the nutrition and exercise road. Another option is to hire a wellness coach who either meets with you in person or talks to you over the phone once a week, helping you design effective strategies to lose weight, exercise, and reduce stress.

A fitness professional can provide something that can be critical in maintaining your fitness routine: accountability. You are likely to be more motivated to keep up your nutrition and fitness program if you're paying someone, and when she is counting on you to show up on time and ready to sweat. What's more, hiring a personal trainer allows you to delegate the responsibility for planning routines to a person with a specific knowledge base—similar to what you may do with certain aspects of your business.

"Having a trainer opens you up to a different paradigm, a new way of exercising," says Glenn Dietzel, a business consultant and CEO of AwakenTheAuthor-Within.com. "They can take you to a level you couldn't get to on your own."

Suzy Jurist—who runs SJI Associates, an advertising and design firm in New York City—works out with a trainer two or three times a week, focusing on exercises that target the core. She began her fitness program after experiencing weight gain with the birth of her children. "If you can afford a trainer," she says, "it's one of the nicest luxuries in life."

Although a trainer can be certified by a private organization, currently there are neither minimum qualifications for calling yourself a personal trainer nor a national standard. Trainers can be found on staff at health facilities and can be hired to come to your home. To find a trainer, check with your club if you belong to one, ask fitness-minded friends for a reference, talk to your doctor, or call a local physical therapist.

You should interview possible trainers to see if they would be a good fit with your personality and goals. In addition to getting an idea of how comfortable you feel with particular trainers, find out some more information:

- How long have they been training clients?
- Can you contact current and former clients?

- Do they participate in ongoing professional training?
- What kind of fitness routine do they themselves follow? If you're planning to train for an event, such as a triathlon, marathon, or long-distance bike ride, it's helpful if the trainer has personal experience.
- Do they have one or more up-to-date certifications from nationally-recognized and accredited organizations, such as the National Academy of Sports Medicine, the American College of Sports Medicine, or the National Strength and Conditioning Association (check for accreditation through the National Commission for Certifying Agencies).
- Are they insured, and do they have current certification in CPR and, if you think it's important, training in first aid and automated external defibrillators?
- What is their relevant academic background, such as a degree in exercise science or kinesiology?
- What is their price, and are there long-term package rates? Fees can vary from $20 to $100 per hour.
- What kind of fitness, health, and goal assessment will they do? For example, will they measure blood pressure and body fat, and help you determine what your short- and long-range goals are? Stay away from trainers who seem to have a "one-size-fits-all" approach.
- What is their policy on cancellations and billing?

◆ ◆ ◆ ◆ ◆

But no matter how good a personal trainer is, ultimately the key to getting in shape is within you and in your ability to constantly improve, something you do every day in your business. You now have knowledge of how to eat well, exercise, and manage your stress, as well as a powerful understanding of the vision that motivates you. With these insights, you'll enjoy the increased self-confidence and sense of control that comes from knowing that you are taking charge of your well-being. And you won't just improve your health and fitness, you'll begin to feel more energy in your work. Most important, in the days and weeks ahead, you'll discover a renewed enthusiasm in every aspect of your life.

> ### *Action* Items
>
> ➤ Sign up for a local athletic event (a 5K running event, for example) in your hometown, scheduled a few months from now.
>
> ➤ If you're planning a vacation in the near future, make it an active trip that includes at least some physical activity while you soak up the local culture.
>
> ➤ If you don't have a gym membership, call a local health club in the coming week to inquire about membership rates and any available personal training packages.

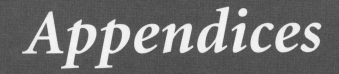

# Appendices

# Starting a Workplace Wellness Program

With health-care costs increasing every year, businesses are frequently turning to workplace wellness programs to help workers get and stay healthy. A 2005–2006 survey of 275 companies found that 41 percent had already launched a health and productivity project as part of an overall health-care strategy, while almost 32 percent intended to start a plan within the year.

Employers are beginning to realize that keeping their workers healthy is good not just for the employees but for the company as a whole. "We want our employees to be healthy and in good shape," says Susan Solovic, CEO and chair of SBTV.com. "That way, they can be even better contributors to the overall goals and objectives of the company. But most important, we want everybody to take care of themselves because we really care about their health."

Research supports the idea that workplace wellness programs decrease absenteeism and health-care costs, according to the American Institute for Preventive Medicine (www.healthylife.com), which works with health-care organizations and corporations to help implement health promotion strategies. As mentioned in Chapter 1, a review of nine big employers found that for every dollar spent on a health program, the savings were from $1.49 to $4.91.

While large companies have access to more resources, it's a little harder for small- and medium-sized companies to squeeze wellness into the budget. But you don't need a lavish company fitness facility if you take creative steps to encourage employees to stay fit. For example, Gini Dietrich owns Arment Dietrich, a growing public relations firm with more than 20 clients. She's a true believer in staying active and eating well, and has made sure she gives her employees time to take care of their own health. She realizes that people who exercise are better, more productive employees. "Because we bill our time," she says, "I give my staff an incentive to exercise by adding a billable job code for their workouts. It counts toward their annual billable goals. I also offer a small gym membership reimbursement."

Dan Santy, founder of Santy Advertising, makes sure to keep nutritious snacks in the office lunchroom for him and his staff. "We're really encouraging a healthy lifestyle," he says. "I firmly believe that the people who are the most active and fit, and who have good healthy diets, don't miss work."

At Stacy's Pita Chip Company, business owners Stacy Madison and Mark Andrus believe having healthy workers makes for a better work environment and a better company. "We try to promote a healthy atmosphere," Madison says. "It's important for us as leaders to show that it's important." Madison and Andrus give each employee a $500 annual benefit to be applied toward anything that is health and fitness related. "It doesn't have to be a gym membership," Madison says. "One person took a dance class. Someone could apply it to a healthy cooking class if they wanted to. It's an incentive for people to start bringing some healthier aspects into their life."

Promoting a companywide wellness mentality keeps people motivated, Madison believes. "A lot of times people will go for a walk together," she says. "One of our employees was trying to quit smoking, so instead of having a cigarette, she would recruit another person to take a walking break. And that was one fewer cigarette that she smoked that day."

If you're contemplating a workplace wellness program, the American Institute for Preventive Medicine recommends including the following elements:

- *Assessment.* As with your own health and fitness, it's a good idea to get a picture of your employees' health status at the beginning of the wellness program. This could include a screening for conditions such as high blood pressure and cholesterol.
- *Communication materials.* Newsletters and paycheck inserts can keep the idea of health and fitness regularly in the minds of employees.
- *Self-help materials.* Workers can learn about quitting smoking and weight loss at their own pace. The information could come in the form of CD-ROMS, audiotapes, and booklets.
- *Low-cost options.* Even if the budget is tight, simple steps can be taken. Measure out a short walking route around the neighborhood and post a map somewhere in the office. Combat employee stress by placing comfortable chairs away from noise and near a radio playing relaxing music. Poll your employees to see if they'd be interested in having a local massage therapist come into the office once a week for inexpensive 15-minute massages they could pay for out of pocket. Buy fresh fruit or healthy snacks for around the office.

# Calories Burned by Activity

Your body burns calories every minute of the day. How much you burn for any given activity depends on a number of factors, including how much of your body is involved, your weight, the type of activity, and your skill at performing it. But this table provides rough estimates of how many calories you burn during a range of pursuits, from exercise to chores to working at your desk. Estimations are standardized to one hour of activity.

The following table is adapted from "Compendium of Physical Activities: An update of activity codes and MET intensities," by B.E. Ainsworth, W.L. Haskell, M.C. Whitt, M.L. Irwin, A.M. Swartz, S.J. Strath, W.L. O'Brien, D.R. Bassett Jr., K.H. Schmitz, P.O. Emplaincourt, D.R. Jacobs Jr., and A.S. Leon, *Medicine and Science in Sports and Exercise*, 2000; 32(Suppl.):S498-S516.

| One Hour of Activity | For a Person Who Weighs: | |
| --- | --- | --- |
| | **130 Pounds** | **180 Pounds** |
| **Cardio** | | |
| Bicycling, 12–13.9 mph, leisurely or moderate effort | 473 | 655 |
| Bicycling, 16–19 mph, very fast | 709 | 982 |
| Bicycling, stationary, moderate effort | 414 | 573 |
| Bicycling, stationary, vigorous effort | 620 | 859 |
| Mountain biking | 502 | 695 |
| Rowing, stationary, moderate effort | 414 | 573 |
| Rowing, stationary, vigorous effort | 502 | 695 |
| Running up stairs | 886 | 1,227 |
| Running, 12 minutes per mile | 473 | 655 |
| Running, 10 minutes per mile | 591 | 818 |
| Running, 8 minutes per mile | 739 | 1,023 |
| Running, 7 minutes per mile | 827 | 1,145 |
| Swimming laps, freestyle, moderate or light effort | 414 | 573 |
| Swimming laps, freestyle, vigorous effort | 591 | 818 |
| Walking, pushing or pulling a stroller with a child | 148 | 205 |
| Walking, up stairs | 473 | 655 |
| Walking, 3 mph, moderate pace, level surface | 195 | 270 |
| Walking, 4.5 mph, brisk pace, level surface | 372 | 515 |
| Walking, 3.5 mph, uphill | 355 | 491 |
| **Resistance Training** | | |
| Weight lifting, light or moderate effort | 177 | 245 |

| One Hour of Activity | For a Person Who Weighs: | |
|---|---|---|
| | 130 Pounds | 180 Pounds |
| **Resistance Training** | | |
| Weight lifting, vigorous effort | 355 | 491 |
| **Recreation** | | |
| Dancing | 266 | 368 |
| Fishing in a stream, in waders | 355 | 491 |
| Ice fishing, sitting | 118 | 164 |
| **Chores** | | |
| Auto repair | 177 | 245 |
| Chopping wood | 355 | 491 |
| Cleaning gutters | 295 | 409 |
| Feeding animals | 148 | 205 |
| Grocery shopping | 136 | 188 |
| Hanging storm windows | 295 | 409 |
| Making your bed | 118 | 164 |
| Moving furniture | 355 | 491 |
| Mowing the lawn | 325 | 450 |
| Operating a snowblower | 266 | 368 |
| Painting | 266 | 368 |
| Shoveling snow | 355 | 491 |
| Sweeping, household | 195 | 270 |
| Vacuuming | 207 | 286 |
| Washing car, vigorous effort | 266 | 368 |
| **Sports/Activities** | | |
| Backpacking | 414 | 573 |
| Basketball | 473 | 655 |

| One Hour of Activity | For a Person Who Weighs: | |
|---|---|---|
| | **130 Pounds** | **180 Pounds** |
| **Sports/Activities** | | |
| Billiards | 148 | 205 |
| Bowling | 177 | 245 |
| Boxing, punching a heavy bag | 355 | 491 |
| Football, touch or flag | 473 | 655 |
| Golf, carrying clubs | 266 | 368 |
| Handball | 709 | 982 |
| Hiking | 355 | 491 |
| Judo, jujitsu, karate, kickboxing, tae kwon do | 591 | 818 |
| Jumping rope, moderate effort | 591 | 818 |
| Kayaking | 295 | 409 |
| Racquetball | 414 | 573 |
| Snorkeling | 295 | 409 |
| Soccer | 414 | 573 |
| Surfing, body or board variety | 177 | 245 |
| Tai chi | 236 | 327 |
| Tennis, singles | 473 | 655 |
| Hatha yoga | 148 | 205 |
| **At Work** | | |
| Bartending | 136 | 188 |
| Carpentry | 207 | 286 |
| Desk work | 89 | 123 |
| Firefighting (climbing ladder with full gear) | 650 | 900 |
| Making photocopies | 136 | 188 |
| Policing (making an arrest) | 236 | 327 |

| One Hour of Activity | For a Person Who Weighs: | |
| --- | --- | --- |
| | 130 Pounds | 180 Pounds |
| **At Work** | | |
| Sitting in a meeting | 89 | 123 |
| Walking around the office at a moderate pace | 195 | 270 |
| **Winter Sports** | | |
| Cross-country skiing, uphill | 975 | 1,350 |
| Cross-country skiing, 4.0–4.9 mph, moderate effort | 473 | 655 |
| Cross-country skiing, 5.0–7.9 mph, vigorous effort | 532 | 736 |
| Curling | 236 | 327 |
| Downhill skiing, moderate effort | 355 | 491 |
| Ice hockey | 473 | 655 |
| Ice skating, 9 mph or less | 325 | 450 |
| Ice skating, more than 9 mph | 532 | 736 |
| Sledding, tobogganing, bobsledding, luge | 414 | 573 |
| Snowmobiling | 207 | 286 |
| Snowshoeing | 473 | 655 |
| **Miscellaneous** | | |
| Gardening | 236 | 327 |
| Reading | 59 | 82 |
| Sex | 77 | 106 |
| Sleeping | 53 | 74 |
| Toweling off after a shower | 118 | 164 |
| Watching television or a movie | 59 | 82 |

# Putting the Taste in Healthy Cooking

If you think you have to sacrifice taste to eat healthy, think again. Chad Luethje—executive chef at Red Mountain Spa, an active-oriented retreat in St. George, Utah—caters to a health-conscious clientele looking for delicious food that meshes with a fitness lifestyle.

"One of the common misconceptions out there is that spa foods consist of miniscule portions of tofu, a little seaweed, and some overcooked, under-seasoned vegetables," says Luethje, who stays active with hiking, mountain biking, and skiing. "It's really not the case."

Luethje keeps his meals healthy by making creative but easy-to-implement alterations that reduce calories, fat, and sodium. He agreed to share some of his culinary secrets to healthy eating at home and when you're dining out.

### Use the Agave Alternative

Luethje's recipes often use agave syrup, a naturally occurring fructose from the agave cactus. "It comes out as a light-colored syrup and has a lighter, honey type of taste," he says. "We use that a lot in our baking and for pancakes or French toast as a low-sugar alternative." Agave is low on the glycemic index,

Luethje explains, which means it does not cause a dramatic rise in your blood sugar levels, helping you maintain a more constant level of energy.

### Keep Soup Light

When making a cream-type soup—such as butternut squash, cream of potato, or asparagus—reduce the fat and calories by cutting out the chicken or veal stocks that typically are used. Instead, use a vegetable stock, which is low in calories and fat. Also, in place of cream or milk, add in extra amounts of the main ingredient (for example, squash or potato) in pureed form. "This acts as both a thickening agent and a flavor enhancer," Luethje says. "It eliminates the need to add cream at all. If you still want more of a creamy texture, try adding soy milk, which gives you some good, healthy proteins."

### Use Kosher Salt

This typically contains zero additives and has larger, coarser crystals than regular table salt. "With Kosher salt, it's easier to watch the amount that you're adding into foods because it's easier to control what you're pinching in," Luethje says. "We also put this in our salt shakers so people really have to work to get it out. Subconsciously we're trying to break them of the habit of adding so much salt."

### Brighten Up Your Food

To cut down on your sodium intake, use a squeeze of citrus or citrus zest from a lemon, lime, or orange. "This is a good, healthful substitute for salt," Luethje says. "It really brightens up the flavors." To make citrus zest, Luethje uses a kitchen tool called a Microplane zester to grate the peel's outermost layer. "We'll just do a quick zest as a garnish over a pasta dish, soup, or a salad," he says.

### Make Your Veggies Healthy

You don't have to drown vegetables in butter, salt, and pepper to enhance flavor. One of Luethje's suggestions: steam them, adding a spritz of extra virgin olive oil, a small pinch of salt, and some fresh chopped herbs. "Grilling is another option," he adds. "You can do a very quick marinade of olive oil, chopped garlic, and a few dried herbs, and just toss the vegetables in that mixture enough to coat the outside." After grilling, you can serve them whole or chop them up for a grilled vegetable salad or as a topping for a pizza.

### Spray It

Use a spray bottle or mister to dispense cooking oils—this allows you to better control amounts. Each pull of the trigger gives you between an eighth and a quarter of a teaspoon of oil, Luethje explains. (But don't use the bottle for storage for more than a few days to avoid the oil taking on the taste of the plastic.)

### Snack Smart

For around-the-house healthy snacks, one of Luethje's favorites is cutting up papaya or mango spears, and tossing them with a squeeze of fresh lime juice and a pinch of chili powder. When on the go, he suggests whole-grain crackers and fresh fruits, especially apples and oranges. "They have a very low glycemic index and are pretty high in fiber," he says. "So they slow the absorption of sugar into your liver, allowing it to enter your blood stream more slowly. This helps you keep a nice even keel, as opposed to those big spikes and valleys that tend to cause people to binge."

# Health and Fitness on the Web

Although the internet is rife with unbounded claims for every manner of health and fitness product, there are numerous web sites that offer excellent information. At your fingertips, you have access to the knowledge of academic and government experts, scholarly journals with the latest research findings, and health advice from national nonprofit organizations. Often, just a few minutes of Google searches and surfing can turn up studies and reports on a topic you're interested in. Of course, you have to consider the source and be wary of financial or other possible biases.

Here are some of the best and most informative sites you'll find.

- *www.americanheart.org and www.strokeassociation.org.* Information on heart disease and stroke, including warning signs, from the American Heart Association and the American Stroke Association.
- *www.cancer.gov.* Coverage of cancer topics from the National Cancer Institute, including information on clinical trials.
- *www.cancer.org.* Information on cancer, including support resources, from the American Cancer Society.

- *www.cdc.gov.* Health information from the Centers for Disease Control and Prevention, including the latest information on avian influenza (bird flu), plus more data and statistics than you ever thought existed.
- *www.diabetes.niddk.nih.gov.* A clearinghouse of diabetes information, including prevention techniques, symptoms, and treatment.
- *www.diabetes.org.* A breakdown of the different types of diabetes, as well as advice on exercise and nutrition (including recipes) from the American Diabetes Association.
- *www.hsph.harvard.edu/nutritionsource.* A web site from the Department of Nutrition of the Harvard School of Public Health with indepth articles on fats, cholesterol, fiber, vitamins, diabetes, and more. Bonus: a helpful article on how to interpret nutrition news.
- *www.mayoclinic.com.* Information on diseases and conditions, a body mass index calculator, and more.
- *www.medlineplus.com.* A medical dictionary and encyclopedia and helpful links to other resources, maintained by the U.S. National Library of Medicine and the National Institutes of Health.
- *www.mypyramid.gov.* The federal government's site for its recently re-issued food guide pyramid, with an interactive tool that personalizes the pyramid's recommendations.
- *www.nal.usda.gov/fnic/foodcomp.* Nutrient breakdowns (for protein, carbs, fat, vitamins, and minerals) of your favorite foods, courtesy of the USDA Agricultural Research Service's Nutrient Data Laboratory.
- *www.ods.od.nih.gov/Health_Information/ODS_Frequently_Asked_Questions .aspx.* Frequently asked questions and fact sheets for dietary supplements from the federal government's Office of Dietary Supplements.
- *www.pubmed.gov.* A database of thousands of journals with studies on health, diet, and exercise—abstracts are free, and many journals also make full-text articles freely available.
- *www.realage.com.* Questions about your health history give you an estimation of your biological age compared with your calendar age (i.e., you may be 50 years old on the calendar, but you're in such good shape that you're actually equivalent biologically to a 38-year-old).

- *www.webmd.com*. Features include health news, health guides, and an interactive symptom checker.
- *www.womenshealth.gov*. A range of health topics for women from the U.S. Department of Health and Human Services; a link to men's health issues is at www.womenshealth.gov/mens.

# Entrepreneur Web Sites

Here is a listing of the web sites of the entrepreneurs featured in this book.

**Terri Alpert**
Uno Alla Volta LLC and Professional Cutlery Direct LLC
*www.cookingenthusiast.com*
*www.unoallavolta.com*

**Mark Andrus and Stacy Madison**
Stacy's Pita Chip Company
*www.pitachips.com*

**Gini Dietrich**
Arment Dietrich
*www.armentdietrich.com*

**Glenn Dietzel**
AwakenTheAuthorWithin.com
*www.AwakenTheAuthorWithin.com*

**Stephen Gatlin**
Gatlin Education Services
*www.gatlineducation.com*
*www.theelearningcenter.com*

**Claire Gruppo**
Gruppo, Levey & Co.
*www.gruppolevey.com*

**Max Hoes**
CFR Line
*www.cfrline.com*

**Suzy Jurist and Dan O'Shea**
SJI Associates
*www.sjiassociates.com*

**Jon Lieb**
Thirty Ink Media & Marketing
*www.30-ink.com*

**Doug MacLean**
Talking Rain
*www.talkingrain.com*

**Jennifer Melton and Brennan Johnson**
Cloud Star
*www.cloudstar.com*

**Margaret Moore**
Wellcoaches Corporation
*www.wellcoaches.com*

**Mike Nagel**
Incisive Surgical
*www.insorb.com*

**Mark Plaatjes**
Boulder Running Company
*www.boulderrunningcompany.com*

**Dominic Rubino**
Fulcrum Agency
*www.fulcrumagency.com*
*www.ultimatesalestips.com*

**Dan Santy**
Santy Advertising
*www.santy.com*

**Brian Scudamore**
1-800-GOT-JUNK?
*www.1800gotjunk.com*

**Robert Smith**
Robert Smith & Associates
*www.bobsmithpr.com*

**Susan Solovic**
SBTV.com (Small Business Television)
*www.sbtv.com*

**Richard Thompson**
The Meow Mix Company
*www.meowmix.com*

**Jim Wilcher**
The Wilcher Group
*www.wilcher.com*

**Kathy Wise, RD**
NutraWise
*www.nutrawise.com*

**Stanley Wunderlich**
Consulting for Strategic Growth 1 Ltd.
*www.cfsg1.com*

# About the Author

Tom Weede is a freelance writer specializing in health and fitness topics. A former senior editor for *Men's Fitness* magazine, he is certified as a Health/Fitness Instructor with the American College of Sports Medicine and is a Certified Strength and Conditioning Specialist with the National Strength and Conditioning Association. He is a member of the National Association of Science Writers and has explored public health issues through the Journalism Boot Camp at the Centers for Disease Control and Prevention. He overcame struggles with his weight by starting a regular running routine in his late 20s, is now an avid runner and cyclist, and has completed several Ironman® triathlons. He lives with his wife, Adrienne, in Oro Valley, Arizona.

# Index